A Handbook
of Traditional
Chinese
Gynecology

A Handbook of Traditional Chinese Gynecology

Compiled by
The Zhejiang College
of Traditional
Chinese Medicine

translated by
Zhang Ting-liang
and
Bob Flaws

Fourth Revised Edition

BLUE POPPY PRESS

Published by:

Blue Poppy Press
3450 Penrose Place, Suite 110
Boulder, CO 80301

Fourth Edition June, 1995
Fifth Printing May, 1998

ISBN 0-936185-06-6

Printed at Maple Vail Book Manufacturing Co.
on acid free, recycled paper.

10 9 8 7 6

COMP Designation: Functional translation

Preface to Fourth Edition

In 1986, I asked Zhang Ting-liang, then working as an English language translator at the Shanghai College of Traditional Chinese Medicine, to select a basic TCM gynecology textbook and translate it for publication in the English. The book he chose was written by Profs. Song Guang-ji and Yu Xiao-zhen of the Zhejiang College of TCM in Hangzhou and was at that time that TCM college's basic gynecology text. Its Chinese title is *Zhong Yi Fu Ke Shou Ce (A Handbook of Traditional Chinese Gynecology)*. It was originally published in China in 1984. Mr. Zhang used the 1985 edition for his translation.

Our first Blue Poppy Press edition of this book appeared in 1987. Since then, it has gone through four revisions, in part because we believe that this book is still the best introduction to TCM gynecology available in English. This book is classified according to the Council of Oriental Medical Publishers (COMP) system of designation as a functional translation. Nevertheless, it uses a standard translational terminology for the main technical terms as they appear in Nigel Wiseman and Ken Boss' *A Glossary of Chinese Medical Terms and Acupuncture Points* published by Paradigm Publications, Brookline, MA, 1990. The main exception to this is that we have used the words network vessels to translate the Chinese *luo* (络) based on revisions supplied to me by Nigel Wiseman.

This revision is the most extensive one we have undertaken on this book to date. It was initiated as part of my preparation for teaching a postgraduate certification class in TCM gynecology. Hopefully, it now reads much closer to the original Chinese than it formerly did. Besides retranslating the entire book, we have also added Pinyin identifications for all the medicinals. The identifications of medicinals in this book are based on Bensky and Gamble's *Chinese Herbal Medicine: Materia Medica*; Cloudburst Press' *A Barefoot Doctor's Manual;* Hong-yen Hsu's *Oriental Materia Medica: A Concise Guide*; Southern Materials Center's reissue of *Chinese Materia Medica*, Vol 1-6; and the Shanghai Science & Technology Press' *Zhong Yao Da Ci Dian (Encyclopedia of Chinese Medicinals)*.

Readers interested in studying TCM gynecology in more depth are referred to my own series of clinical manuals on this specialty. This consists of *My Sister the Moon: The Diagnosis & Treatment of Menstrual Diseases by Traditional Chinese Medicine; Fire in the Valley: The TCM Diagnosis & Treatment of Vaginal Diseases; Path of Pregnancy, Vol. I: A Handbook of Traditional Chinese Gestational & Birthing Diseases; Path of Pregnancy, Vol. II: A Handbook of Traditional Chinese Postpartum Diseases; Fulfilling the Essence: A Handbook of Traditional & Contemporary Chinese Treatments for Female Infertility;* and *PMS: Its Cause, Diagnosis & Treatment According to Traditional Chinese Medicine.* In addition, readers are also referred to Blue Poppy Press' translation of *Fu Qing Zhu Nu Ke (Fu Qing-zhu's Gynecology)*, the single most important premodern Chinese gynecology text. As the reader will see, more formulas in this book have been taken from that book than any other.

Bob Flaws
Mar. 6, 1995

Contents

Chapter One

The Physiological Characteristics of Females

Women have a female wrapper (*nu zi bao*), also called the fetal palace or uterus (*zi gong*), as well as other reproductive organs. The uterus is located in the very center of the lower abdomen, between the urinary bladder and the rectum. It is connected to the wrapper network vessels (*bao luo*), the wrapper vessel (*bao mai*), the birth canal, the genitalia, and the other reproductive organs. In the *Nei Jing (Inner Classic)*, it is called an extraordinary bowel. It governs menstruation and pregnancy. The uterus is categorized as an extraordinary bowel because it neither pertains to a particular viscera or bowel nor does it share an interior/exterior relationship with any internal organ. Nevertheless, the uterus is closely related to the qi and blood, viscera and bowels, and the channels and network vessels of the entire body.

Women's physiology is characterized by the menstrual flow, vaginal discharge, pregnancy, and birthing. Women are also especially liable to damage of the blood. The generation, circulation, and control of the blood depend upon the engenderment, transformation, regulation, and discipline of the qi. Conversely, the qi must be enriched and nourished by the blood. Thus it is said that, "Qi is the commander of the blood, while blood is the mother of qi." Because of the interdependence of qi and blood, a woman's good health depends upon the well-coordinated regulation and harmony of the qi and blood. Both the qi and blood originate from the viscera and bowels. The heart controls the blood. The liver stores the blood. The spleen contains the blood. The kidneys store the essence, and the essence transforms the blood. The lungs control the qi, and the qi commands the blood. In addition, the spleen and stomach are known as the source of qi and blood engenderment and transformation. Therefore, only when the five viscera function in peace and harmony can the qi and blood flow freely and easily. This then leads to the sea of blood being full and exuberant. Fullness leads to spillage and the menstruation comes normally. In this case, gestational and birthing diseases are not easily engendered. The above are the essential points relating to female physiology and their relationship to the viscera and bowels and qi and blood. Among the viscera and bowels, the kidneys, spleen, liver, and heart are the most important.

The functions of the channels and network vessels consist of transporting and moving the qi and blood and connecting the viscera and bowels above and below so as to function synergistically, thus making the body a single organic unit. In particular, female physiology is closely related to the channels and network vessels: the extraordinary vessels of the *chong, ren, du,* and *dai,* as well as the foot *shao yin* kidney channel, foot *jue yin* liver channel, foot *tai yin* spleen channel, and foot *yang ming* stomach channel. Of these, the *chong* and *ren* vessels are the most important. Wang Bing, a physician of the Tang Dynasty, said:

> "The *ren mai* and *chong mai* are extraordinary channels. When kidney qi is wholly exuberant, the *chong* and *ren* flow freely. The menstrual blood increases and is exuberant and correspondingly descends periodically. The *chong* is known as the sea of blood, while the *ren mai* governs the uterus and fetus (*bao tai*). When these two mutually promote each other, one is able to have a child.

The *Nei Jing (Inner Classic)* says, "The *ren mai* is free flowing, the *tai chong mai* is exuberant, and the menstruation descends periodically..." These words illustrate that the *chong* and *ren* are of fundamental importance in the reproductive functions of females. This is why, when speaking of obstetrical and gynecological complaints, often it is said that these channels are responsible for the generations of posterity without reference to the viscera and bowels.

Anatomically, the *chong* and *ren* originate from the uterus. The *ren mai* governs all the yin of the body, while the *chong mai* functions as the sea of the twelve regular channels. As for the *du mai,* the sea of all yang, it also

2

originates from the uterus from which it ascends along the spinal column. When yang engenders, yin grows, and the two vessels of the *ren* and *du* mutually pass into one another. Thus the *du mai* also plays an important role in female physiology. As the *Nei Jing (Inner Classic)* says, "When the *du mai* is diseased...women cannot conceive." As far as the *dai mai* is concerned, it restricts the *chong, ren,* and *du* channels by encircling the lumbar region. It is believed that the *chong, ren,* and *du mai* share the same origin but diverge and follow each their own course. But all are bound by the *dai mai.* Furthermore, network vessels distributed throughout the uterus connect upward with the heart and downward with the kidneys respectively. In addition, their relationship with the internal organs is further strengthened not only by the convergence of the three channels of the liver, spleen, and kidney at the *ren* channel but also by the concentration of their minor network vessels in the genitalia. In sum, the uterus is deeply involved with the condition of the viscera and bowels, the qi and blood, and the channels and network vessels in general and with the *chong, ren,* liver, spleen, and kidney channels in particular. This is in spite of the common terminology of extraordinary organ which might otherwise imply a solitary organ disconnected from and discretionary to the rest of the body.

Section One

The Menstrual Cycle

In healthy females, menstruation begins on a regular monthly cycle at around 14 years of age. This cycle should be approximately 28 days in length. Menarche is believed to be related to the fullness and sufficiency of the kidney qi and the exuberance of the *chong* and *ren* vessels. It is pointed out in the *Su Wen (Simple Questions)* that:

> The *tian gui* arrives at the age of 14 if the *ren mai* is free-flowing and the *tai chong mai* is exuberant. The menstruation descends periodically, and thus one can have children... At 7x7, the *ren mai* is vacuous and the *tai chong mai* is debilitated and scanty. The *tian gui* is exhausted and the

3

pathways are not free-flowing. Thus the body is decrepit and there are no children.

Chen Zi-ming says:

> The *chong* is the sea of blood and the *ren* governs the *bao tai*. If these two vessels are flowing freely, the menstrual blood increases and is exuberant. Correspondingly, it periodically descends, normally 1 time every 3x10 days.

In the term *tian gui*, *tian* refers to the heavenly true qi and *gui* refers to *ren* and *gui* of water (*i.e.*, the two of the ten heavenly stems relating to water). This also means that kidney water is the root of the body and its function. When a woman reaches approximately the age of 14, her kidney water is full and sufficient. This enables the *ren* to flow unobstructedly to her uterus. It indicates the beginning of a woman's prime when her sea of blood/*chong mai* is exuberant. Therefore, her menstrual blood is so full and exuberant that it brims over periodically. However, when the *ren mai* and *chong mai* become vacuous and kidney water is almost debilitated at the age of 7x7 or 49, menopause takes place and a woman's reproductive capacity declines. Menarche may range widely from 12-18 years of age because of the variability in individual constitutions and in local climates. In most cases, menstruation is expected to return monthly after its first appearance. However, in some women, it may be delayed as long as from 1-2 months or even up to 6 months after its first appearance. If a maiden has no other complaint than that her second period is overdue, clinically she is considered normal even though she may be embarrassed by the temporary absence of her menses. Such a delay is because the menstrual blood will not flow regularly until the kidney qi becomes full and exuberant as a woman becomes more mature. In the same way, the arrival of the climacteric can also be influenced by one's general constitution and the climate and may occur earlier or later.

The normal menstrual cycle is about 28 days in length. However, it is also considered normal if it arrives between 25-35 days. The menstrual discharge itself usually lasts for 3-5 days, with some exceptional cases lasting 7 days. The menstrual volume for the unmarried (*i.e.*, virgin) is normally about 50-100ml in total. It is often more than this in married (*i.e.*, sexually active) women. The menstrual blood is usually relatively light in color at the onset and darkens during the following days. The normal menstrual discharge should be free from clots and specific odor and be neither watery nor sticky.

In most women, a series of changes, such as slight soreness in the low back region, lower abdominal distention, weakness of the limbs, dizziness, and breast distention, may be felt just prior to or during the period. These usually disappear spontaneously upon the completion of the period.

Bimonthly, quarterly, and even annual menstruation do occur normally in some women simply due to differences in constitution. The absence of menstruation during one's entire lifetime accompanied by the ability to conceive is called occult menstruation. The regular arrival of the period during pregnancy without the slightest injury to the fetus is called stimulated menstruation, flourishing fetus, or dirty fetus. Although these two conditions are rarely encountered, they are not considered abnormal.

Section Two

Pregnancy & Parturition

Pregnancy takes place in females upon the fertilization of the ovum. According to Western medicine, conception is the result of the union of sperm and ovum in the area of the ampulla of the uterine tube after the maturation of the reproductive organs. The physiological mechanism of the fallopian tube pushes the zygote into the cavity of the uterus where it implants in the endometrium and grows steadily into a fetus.

Pregnancy is typically accompanied by a series of physiological changes which cause the suspension of the menses, an increase in vaginal excreta, a change in the pigmentation of the external genitalia, the enlargement of the breasts which evolves from slight distention, and the darkening of the

5

nipples and areolar rings. In some women, a small amount of lacteal discharge can be expressed during the early stages of pregnancy. This is called initial lactation. Most expectant mothers develop a craving for sour foods and a concomitant distaste for other foods and flavors. There may also be nausea, vomiting, or dizziness. This is called *e zu* or morning sickness (literally, malign obstruction; connotatively, nausea due to obstruction). These symptoms usually subside spontaneously by the end of the first trimester. However, these symptoms may persist beyond this length of time. Enlargement of the lower abdomen is usually not evident until at least 3 months after conception. Later still, the woman will typically experience a subjective feeling of the fetus' movement. Frequent urination and constipation are typical complaints during the last trimester, with the growth of the fetus putting more noticeable pressure on the bladder and rectum.

The pregnant woman is advised to modify both her mental/emotional outlook and her lifestyle in order to ensure the healthy development of her baby. This is called fetal education. Fetal education refers to the adoption of educational measures in order to cultivate the fetus during the course of their uterine development. This idea is actually quite scientific and conforms not only to the theory of prenatal care but also to the goal of raising the standard of health of the people. The *Shi Ji (Historical Records)* tells a story in which the mother of the first emperor of the Western Zhou dynasty refused to look upon adverse colors or to hear indecent sounds or the utterance of any arrogant words. Because of this, she bore a son who achieved great accomplishments later when he came to power. This is the earliest historical reference to the practice of fetal education. Later on, more explicit comments were made by medical professionals of different dynasties. For example, in the Northern Song, Xu Zi-chai's *Shi Yue Yang Tai Fa (Methods for Nourishing the Fetus in the Ten Months)* and the *Fu Ren Da Quan Liang Fang (A Great Complete [Collection of] Fine Formulas for Women)*, a separate section was specially included entitled fetal education. Briefly, fetal education requires strict regimentation of both one's mental and daily activities from the moment of conception. In terms of daily activity, the expectant mother is suggested to abstain from random use of medications, all alcohol, reckless treatment by acupuncture and

6

moxibustion, lifting heavy objects, climbing heights, and taking other such risks. It was also realized back at that time that a difficult labor is likely to arise from fright and that an infant exposed to fright in utero is more susceptible to epilepsy after birth. In addition, expectant mothers are advised to take frequent leisurely walks and neither to sleep too much nor to become excessively fatigued. Moreover, it is essential that one should abstain from the seven affects, the five unfavorable tastes, and sexual activity.

As for appropriate mental activity, this is described in the *Fu Ren Da Quan Liang Fang (A Great Complete [Collection of] Fine Formulas for Women)* which says:

> The child during the first trimester is called the initial fetus. This is the period during which the infant begins to be molded. If a dignified and elegant stature is desired, the mother should think, speak, and act discreetly. If a handsome offspring is wanted, she should wear a piece of jade. If a witty offspring is desired, she should read verses and poems. This is because the exterior reception communicates with the interior plasticity.

It is also pointed out in the *Zhu Lin Shi Nu Ke (The Bamboo Forest Master's Gynecology)* that:

> Fetal education means remaining tranquil and still. If the qi is regulated, the fetus will be quiet. If the qi counterflows, the fetus will be diseased. The slightest anger will cause qi hinderance and lack of normal or correct flow. Liver qi will thrust upward, causing vomiting and epistaxis...Liver qi will pour downward and cause uterine bleeding and abnormal vaginal discharge. There will be slippery fetus and miscarriage. Therefore, the most important thing the mother should maintain is a stable and smooth circulation of qi so that the infant may gain a bright and cheerful disposition and be free from a surly personality.

The above theories illustrate the profound understanding of fetal education in ancient China. Since family planning is nowadays encouraged and practiced world-wide, these theories are meaningful for us to understand in order to popularize the theory of eugenics.

Being a normal physiological process, parturition is expected about 280 days after conception without induction. The saying that "when a melon is ripe, it falls off the vine" is a vivid description of this process. Paroxysmal contraction of the abdomen, especially a sagging, heavy sensation in the lower abdomen, characterizes the first stage of labor. The more the uterus contracts, the more intense the sagging, heavy sensation in the lumbar and abdominal areas becomes, with decreasingly prolonged intervals in between. The rhythmic contraction of the uterus may be so forceful that the patient feels a pressing need to urinate and/or defecate. Normally, it is the infant's head which makes the first appearance after the full effacement of the cervix. The delivery ends with the recurrence of uterine contractions about 10-15 minutes after delivery of the infant. This is accompanied by vaginal bleeding and the expulsion of the placenta. Therefore, the entire course of delivery includes the time from which the uterus begins regular contractions up until the placenta is completely expelled from the body. Fourteen to 18 hours and 8-12 hours are typically required respectively for primiparas and multiparas.

After delivery, as a result of overexertion and bleeding during delivery, the yin blood in the woman's body may be vacuous and her fluids and humors insufficient. Yin vacuity is not able to subdue yang. Yang qi thus easily floats and scatters. The interstices are not densely packed. A few days after delivery, light fever, aversion to cold, and profuse perspiration may follow and the pulse may be felt to be slow and relaxed or slightly rapid. Medical treatment need not be employed unless these symptoms persist for a number of days. The lochia will come to a pause by itself after tapering off for 7-10 days. It begins bright red in color and later becomes pink. Some women may have bouts of lower abdominal pain due to uterine contraction. This is called "infant pillow pain." This phenomenon is usually self-limiting 1-2 weeks after delivery.

The reestablishment of the menstrual flow after childbirth depends upon whether one breastfeeds or not. Non-breastfeeding women may restore their menstrual cycle in 1-2 months after delivery, whereas those women who breastfeed the baby may regain their periods 6-12 months later.

Chapter Two

A Synopsis of Gynecological Pathology

The *chong, ren, du,* and *dai mai* are the vessels most often involved in gynecological pathophysiology. Diverging from a single source, the *chong, ren,* and *du* are connected with each other by the *dai mai*. It is known that the *ren mai* governs the yin of the entire body and also rules the uterus and fetus, whereas the *chong mai* serves as the sea of blood. Therefore, both are vitally important to both the engenderment of blood and fastening of the fetus. Consequently, damage and detriment of the *chong* and *ren* is believed to be the main cause of gynecological disorders. Direct causes of damage and detriment to the *chong* and *ren* include evil toxin infections and undisciplined bedroom affairs. These may result in either profuse abnormal vaginal discharge or uterine bleeding. Indirect causes of damage and detriment to the *chong* and *ren* include internal damage by the seven affects, invasion by the six external environmental excesses, and loss of discipline in food and drink, each of which may cause disharmony of the qi and blood and loss of regulation of the viscera and bowels.

Emotional disturbances are a major disease cause in gynecology, often resulting in liver qi depression and binding, with blood eventually being affected by qi stagnation. This may lead to the arising of delayed menstruation, painful menstruation, or menstrual block. Emotional disturbances may also result in hyperactivity of liver yang which may lead to the arising of pre-eclampsia and eclampsia. Liver effulgence/blood heat may lead to the arising of profuse uterine bleeding or dribbling and dripping or to menstrual movement hemoptysis or epistaxis. In addition, worry and excessive thought may cause detriment to the heart and spleen. This may lead to amenorrhea or fetal leakage. Fright and fear may damage the kidneys and may lead to miscarriage.

Among the six environmental excesses, cold, heat, and dampness are the foremost in causing gynecological disorders. If the blood is invaded by heat, it moves. If it obtains cold, it congeals. Therefore, heat exuberance can force the blood to move recklessly, leading to the arising of early menstruation, excessive menstruation, and uterine bleeding. If cold is exuberant, it may easily cause painful menstruation, delayed menstruation, or, if severe, concretions and conglomerations. Damp evils invading the spleen may assail the *chong* and *ren*, leading to the arising of abnormal vaginal discharge, uterine bleeding, and irregular menstruation.

Loss of discipline in food and drink may lead to the spleen and stomach's loss of regulation. The source of engenderment and transformation in that case becomes insufficient and the sea of blood consequently empty and vacuous. This can lead to delayed menstruation, scanty menstruation, and menstrual block. If the spleen loses its restraint and containment of the blood, blood follows qi fall. This may lead to excessive menstruation and uterine bleeding. If spleen yang does not transport, dampness and turbidity will pour downward, resulting in abnormal vaginal discharge. All the above indirect causes may lead to dysfunction of the viscera and bowels and disharmony of the qi and blood. Either of these two may cause detriment to the *chong* and *ren* and thus the onset of disease.

Qi and blood are the enrichment and engenderment of the viscera and bowels. Women's menstruation, pregnancy, birthing, and lactation are all the result of the function of the blood. Therefore, the blood in women is easily consumed and damaged, thus leading to insufficiency of blood. In that case, qi has a surplus. However, because the qi and blood are mutually dependent and mutually engender each other, if evils damage the blood, eventually this will affect the qi. Conversely, if the qi aspect suffers disease, the blood will likewise eventually be influenced. Therefore, in order to make a correct differential diagnosis, attention should be paid to the discrimination of the primary etiology causing imbalance of the qi and blood.

Diseases of the blood include blood vacuity, blood stasis, blood heat, and blood cold. Qi diseases consist of qi vacuity, qi stagnation, and qi depression. In clinical practice, blood aspect diseases and qi aspect diseases usually manifest in tandem. If women do not follow the prohibitions regarding sex during menstruation, pregnancy, and postpartum, this can cause damage to the *chong* and *ren*. Clinically, gynecological conditions such as uterine bleeding, slippery fetus, miscarriage, infertility, abnormal vaginal discharge, and concretions and conglomerations are related to detriment and damage of the *chong* and *ren*.

Physiologically, the *chong* and *ren* vessels are intimately related to the liver and kidneys since the liver rules the storage of the blood and the *chong mai* serves as the sea of blood. If the sea of blood stores up and spills over normally and is sufficient, this is the essential cause for the liver to be regular and disciplined. The kidneys are the root of the *chong* and *ren*. It is necessary for the kidney qi to be exuberant for the *ren mai* to be free-flowing, for the *tai chong mai* to be exuberant, and for the menstruation to descend periodically. The liver and kidneys share a common source, and both control the lower burner. This is what is meant by the classical statement, "The eight vessels pertain to the liver and kidneys." Therefore, if the liver and kidneys are insufficient or lose their regularity, this may cause the appearance of the clinical signs and symptoms of detriment and damage of the *chong* and *ren*.

The analysis and discrimination of gynecological disorders is commonly outlined as follows: Early menstruation is due to heat, whereas delayed menstruation is due to cold. Excessive volume pertains to repletion and heat, while scanty volume pertains to vacuity and cold. Profuse uterine bleeding is due to qi vacuity not being able to contain the blood, while dribbling precipitation is due to blood not gathering in the channels. Amenorrhea is divided into blood withering and blood stagnation. In dysmenorrhea, if there is abdominal pain before menstruation, this is mostly due to qi stagnation. If there is abdominal pain after the menstruation, it is mostly due to blood vacuity. Premenstrual epistaxis and hemoptysis are commonly due to blood heat reckless movement. Menstrual movement breast distention and pain are mostly due to liver depression/qi stagnation. Menopausal syndrome is mostly ascribed to kidney vacuity due

11

to aging, qi and blood deficiency detriment, and liver yang harassing above.

Abnormal vaginal discharge is due to disease of the *dai mai*. It is mostly due to spleen vacuity dampness and turbidity pouring downward. Vaginal discharge is divided into five colors of *dai*: green, yellow, red, white, and black. However, in clinical practice, mostly white *dai* and yellow *dai* are seen. Occasionally, one may also see red *dai*. Their pathophysiology is mostly *ren mai* vacuity detriment, *dai mai* loss of restraint, spleen dampness and wind evils invading the wrapper network vessels (*bao luo*). These result in damp heat pouring downward and thus the production of this disease. It may also be caused by direct invasion of evil toxins. These are typically also categorized as damp heat. Zhu Dan-xi says that abnormal vaginal discharge which is red pertains to blood, and white pertains to the qi aspect. In clinical practice, abnormal vaginal discharge which is watery and clear is due to vacuity. Vaginal discharge which is yellow and pasty is due to damp heat. If colored red, it is mixed with heat. Green and black *dai* are seldom seen.

After conception, various diseases may develop. For example, if fetal qi surges upward, this may cause nausea, vomiting, and disgust for food. Water qi damp evils may damage the spleen and stomach and can cause the body to have fetal swelling (*i.e.*, edema) and fetal fullness. Blood vacuity may contract wind, and liver yang may harass above. These may cause the onset of pre-eclampsia. Qi and blood insufficiency of the *chong* and *ren* with consequent damage and detriment commonly cause fetal leakage and miscarriage. These are the most commonly encountered diagnoses for the above gestational disorders. However, individual cases may involve more complicated scenarios and, therefore, require more careful analysis and consideration.

In terms of postpartum diseases, the *Jin Gui Yao Lue (Essentials from the Golden Cabinet)* describes the most commonly seen diseases. For instance, it says:

> Recently delivered women have three diseases: 1) tremors, 2) fainting,

and 3) difficult defecation...If recently postpartum women are blood vacuous, there will be excessive perspiration and susceptibility to wind stroke. Therefore there is tremor disease. If there is perished blood, there is recurrent sweating and excessive cold. Therefore there is fainting. If there is perished fluids and humors with stomach dryness, therefore there is difficult defecation.

In terms of other commonly seen diseases, postpartum lochia stasis and binding causes lower abdominal replete pain. Greatly excessive blood loss causes lower abdomen vacuity pain. If qi does not contain the blood and blood does not gather in the channels, this may cause postpartum uterine bleeding. If qi and blood are both deficient and the constructive and defensive are not harmonious, this can cause postpartum fever. In addition, if postpartum the spleen and stomach are vacuous and weak, lying down and sleeping too much and overeating constructing and nourishing foods may easily cause food damage. While qi vacuity and downward fall with loss of restraint of the wrapper vessel (*bao mai*) may lead to downward desertion of the uterus.

As for the pathophysiology of breast disease, Zhu Dan-xi says:

> The breast is canalized by the *yang ming* and the *jue yin* homes to the nipple. Lactation is quite a delicate function and it can become disharmonious, unregulated, and unnourished due to indignation and anger causing counterflow, depression and oppression causing checking, and thick flavors causing brewing. In that case, the *jue yin* qi does not move. Therefore the portals are not open and the breast milk cannot obtain exit. *Yang ming* heat boils and soars. Heat qi blows. Thus nodules and kernels are engendered which become breast *yong* or abscesses.

Postpartum scanty lactation is due to the mother's body being debilitated and weak and construction and nourishment (*i.e.*, nutrition) not being good. It is also possible for worry and anxiety, indignation and anger to cause depression and oppression. Thus scanty lactation may also be due to essence spirit or mental-emotional causes.

Spasm= wind
Fainting = cold

Constipation - dry heat

13

As described above, it is essential to analyze the disease causes and disease mechanisms of the most commonly seen gynecological patterns and diseases. Because our national medicine (*i.e.*, TCM) stresses the interdependence of the human organism and its surrounding environment, intensive analysis and discrimination of patterns based on the four examinations, the eight principles, qi and blood, viscera and bowels, and channels and network vessels cannot be overemphasized even in the treatment of such seemingly localized disorders discussed above.

Chapter Three

Key Points in the Treatment Methods of Gynecological Diseases

Gynecological disorders are closely related to the whole constitution even though their manifestations appear in the reproductive organs. Therefore, it is necessary to use the four examinations and eight principles to clearly distinguish the viscera from the bowels, the qi from the blood, and the channels and network vessels. In addition, geographical environment, climate, age, general constitution, dietary habits, and individual idiosyncracies should all be taken into account when making a comprehensive pattern discrimination. Thus one will be able to achieve good results. In clinical practice, gynecological diseases are usually linked with the so-called miscellaneous diseases of internal medicine. Within vacuity, there may be repletion. Within repletion, there may be vacuity. Consequently, at the time of treatment, it is very important to clearly distinguish the root from the branch and to use the following therapeutic principles flexibly.

1. Regulating the Qi & Blood

Regulation and harmonization of the qi and blood result in quiet and harmony of the five viscera, free and smooth flow of the channels and network vessels, and fullness and exuberance of the *chong* and *ren*. Thus menstrual diseases, abnormal vaginal discharge, and pre- and postpartum diseases are healed spontaneously and easily.

In using the method of regulating the qi and blood, first one must discriminate where the disease is located, whether in the qi or in the blood.

Because the qi and blood are both so closely related, regulation of the qi and regulation of the blood cannot be separated. Therefore, if disease is located in the qi aspect, one should mainly rectify the qi, assisted by nourishing the blood. If the disease is located in the blood aspect, one should mainly treat the blood, aided by rectifying the qi. The combination of these principles should be regularly followed in order to prevent overdosage of enriching, slimy ingredients when nourishing the blood, and consuming and scattering when rectifying the qi. If there is simultaneous qi vacuity and blood stasis, one should use the supplementing the qi method aided by quickening the blood and transforming stasis ingredients. Similarly, if blood vacuity is accompanied by qi stagnation, one should use the blood-supplementing method assisted by medicinals for moving the qi. Thus one can supplement vacuity without aggravating stagnant evils and attack evils without damaging the righteous.

Commonly Used Medicinals for Regulating the Qi & Blood:

A) Qi-supplementing medicinals: Radix Panacis Ginseng (*Ren Shen*), Radix Codonopsis Pilosulae (*Dang Shen*), Radix Astragali Membranacei (*Huang Qi*), Radix Pseudostellariae (*Tai Zi Shen*), Rhizoma Atractylodis Macrocephalae (*Bai Zhu*), etc.

B) Qi-downbearing medicinals: Lignum Dalbergiae Odoriferae (*Jiang Xiang*), Lignum Aquilariae Agallochae (*Chen Xiang*), Flos Inulae (*Xuan Fu Hua*), Haematitum (*Dai Zhe Shi*), etc.

C) Depression-resolving, qi-moving medicinals: Rhizoma Cyperi Rotundi (*Xiang Fu*), Fructus Citri Seu Ponciri (*Zhi Ke*), Fructus Meliae Toosendan (*Chuan Lian Zi*), Radix Linderae Strychnifoliae (*Wu Yao*), Pericarpium Citri Reticulatae (*Chen Pi*), Pericarpium Viridis Citri Reticulatae (*Qing Pi*), Fructus Citri Sacrodactylis (*Fo Shou*), Flos Rosa Rugosae (*Mei Gui Hua*), Flos Citri Aurantii (*Dai Dai Hua*), Caulis Perillae Frutescentis (*Su Gen*), etc.

D) Blood-supplementing medicinals: Radix Angelicae Sinensis (*Dang Gui*), Gelatinum Corii Asini (*E Jiao*), Radix Albus Paeoniae

Lactiflorae (*Bai Shao*), raw Radix Rehmanniae (*Sheng Di*), prepared Radix Rehmanniae (*Shu Di*), Radix Polygoni Multiflori (*He Shou Wu*), Fructus Lycii Chinensis (*Gou Qi Zi*), etc.

E) Blood-moving, stasis-expelling medicinals: Semen Pruni Persicae (*Tao Ren*), Flos Carthami Tinctorii (*Hong Hua*), Radix Ligustici Wallichii (*Chuan Xiong*), Radix Salviae Miltiorrhizae (*Dan Shen*), Herba Leonuri Heterophylli (*Yi Mu Cao*), Herba Lycopi Lucidi (*Ze Lan*), Rhizoma Sparganii (*San Leng*), Rhizoma Curcumae Zedoariae (*E Zhu*), Semen Vaccariae Segetalis (*Wang Bu Liu Xing*), Pollen Typhae (*Pu Huang*), Feces Trogopterori Seu Pteromi (*Wu Ling Zhi*), Herba Angelicae Anomalae (*Liu Ji Nu*), Fructus Crataegi (*Shan Zha*), etc.

F) Heat-clearing, blood-cooling medicinals: Cornu Rhinocerotis (*Xi Jiao*, substitute Cornu Bubali [*Shui Niu Jiao*]), raw Radix Rehmanniae (*Sheng Di,*) Radix Lithospermi Seu Arnebiae (*Zi Cao*), Cortex Radicis Moutan (*Dan Pi*), Radix Rubiae Cordifoliae (*Qian Cao*), etc.

2. Harmonizing the Spleen & Stomach

The spleen and stomach are the latter heaven or postnatal root and the source of engenderment and transformation. The *chong mai* is connected to the foot *yang ming* stomach channel. If spleen and stomach function loses its regulation, this affects the normal engenderment and transformation of the qi and blood and can lead to *chong* and *ren* detriment and damage and hence to various types of gynecological diseases. The method of fortifying the spleen and harmonizing the stomach is composed of several different principles: for vacuity, supplement; for accumulation, disperse; for cold, warm; and for heat, clear. It is not appropriate to overuse either enriching and slimy or bitter, cold ingredients so as to avoid causing detriment and damage to the spleen and stomach and the righteous qi. For instance, if the spleen loses its fortification and transportation, water dampness stops and gathers. In that case, it is appropriate to use the method of fortifying the spleen and disinhibiting dampness. If the spleen and

17

stomach are regulated and harmonious, then diseases will automatically be cured. In the treatment of gynecological diseases, it is necessary to pay close attention to this.

Commonly Used Medicinals for Harmonizing the Stomach & Spleen:

A) Spleen-supplementing, stomach-fortifying medicinals: Radix Codonopsis Pilosulae (*Dang Shen*), Rhizoma Atractylodis Macrocephalae (*Bai Zhu*), Radix Dioscoreae Oppositae (*Shan Yao*), Semen Euryalis Ferocis (*Qian Shi*), Semen Dolichoris Lablabis (*Bian Dou*), Fructus Zizyphi Jujubae (*Da Zao*), etc.

B) Warming & transporting the spleen & stomach: dried Rhizoma Zingiberis (*Gan Jiang*), fresh Rhizoma Zingiberis (*Sheng Jiang*), Fructus Evodiae Rutecarpae (*Wu Zhu Yu*), ginger(-processed) Rhizoma Pinelliae Ternatae (*Jiang Ban Xia*), Fructus Amomi (*Sha Ren*), Fructus Cardamomi (*Kou Ren*), Flos Caryophylli (*Ding Xiang*), etc.

C) Stomach heat-clearing medicinals: Radix Scutellariae Baicalensis (*Huang Qin*), Rhizoma Coptidis Chinensis (*Huang Lian*), Caulis In Taeniis Bambusae (*Zhu Ru*), Fructus Gardeniae Jasminoidis (*Zhi Zi*), Rhizoma Phragmitis Communis (*Lu Gen*), etc.

D) Stomach yin-nourishing medicinals: Radix Glehniae Littoralis (*Sha Shen*), Herba Dendrobii (*Shi Hu*), Tuber Ophiopogonis Japonicae (*Mai Dong*), Rhizoma Polygonati Odorati (*Yu Zhu*), etc.

E) Accumulation-dispersing, stomach-opening medicinals: Fructus Crataegi (*Shan Zha*), Endothelium Corneum Gigeriae Galli (*Ji Nei Jin*), Fructus Germinatus Oryzae Sativae (*Gu Ya*), Fructus Germinatus Hordei Vulgaris (*Mai Ya*), Massa Medica Fermentata (*Shen Qu*), etc.

F) Spleen-fortifying, dampness-disinhibiting medicinals: Sclerotium Poriae Cocos (*Fu Ling*), Semen Coicis Lachryma-jobi (*Mi Ren*), Rhizoma Atractylodis (*Cang Zhu*), Sclerotium Rubrum Poriae Cocos

(*Chi Ling*), Rhizoma Alismatis (*Ze Xie*), Rhizoma Dioscoreae Hypoglaucae (*Chuan Bi Xie*), Medulla Tetrapanacis Papyriferi (*Tong Cao*), etc.

3. Nourishing the Liver & Kidneys and Boosting the *Chong & Ren*

The liver and kidneys' role in female physiology has been discussed above. One governs storage of the blood and the other governs storage of the essence. Both are connected with the uterus. The liver is the son of the kidneys. The kidneys are the mother of the liver. The liver governs coursing and discharge, while the kidneys govern closure and storage. Thus these two are interdependent and interpromoting. Moreover, this mutual connection between the liver and kidneys is further strengthened through their respective connections with the *ren mai* in the lower abdomen and with a branch of the *chong mai* originating at *Qi Chong* (St 30) on the stomach channel. The *chong mai* overlaps with the foot *shao yin* kidney channel and ascends on either side of the umbilicus. Therefore, conditions of the liver and kidneys and the *chong* and *ren* vessels can be transmitted mutually between each other. Therapeutically, medicinals for nourishing the liver and kidneys can also be used to boost the *chong* and *ren*. When treating based on the above principles, for yin vacuity of the liver and kidneys, it is appropriate to supplement yin. For yang vacuity of the liver and kidneys, it is appropriate to warm and nourish. When the liver and kidneys obtain nourishment, the *chong* and *ren* are regulated and harmonized and consequently, diseases are easily eliminated.

Commonly Used Medicinals for Nourishing the Liver & Kidneys and Boosting the *Chong & Ren*:

A) Liver/kidney yin deficiency medicinals: Prepared Radix Rehmanniae (*Shu Di*), Fructus Corni Officinalis (*Shan Zhu Yu*), Gelatinum Corii Asini (*E Jiao*), Fructus Lycii Chinensis (*Gou Qi Zi*), Plastrum Testudinis (*Gui Ban*), Placenta Hominis (*Zi He Che*), Radix Albus

19

Paeoniae Lactiflorae (*Bai Shao*), Fructus Mori Albi (*Sang Shen*), Fructus Ligustri Lucidi (*Nu Zhen Zi*), Herba Ecliptae Prostrate (*Han Lian Cao*), etc.

B) Kidney yang warming & nourishing medicinals: Cornu Cervi (*Lu Jiao*), Semen Cuscutae (*Tu Si Zi*), Radix Morindae Officinalis (*Ba Ji Tian*), Rhizoma Cibotii Barometz (*Gou Ji*), Herba Cistanchis (*Rou Cong Rong*), Herba Epimedii (*Xian Ling Pi*), Radix Dipsaci (*Xu Duan*), Herba Cynomorii Songarici (*Suo Yang*), Cortex Cinnamomi (*Rou Gui*), etc.

In conclusion, enriching and nourishing the liver and kidneys is the source of boosting the *chong* and *ren*. When the source is exuberant, essence blood is full and disease automatically is healed.

The treatment methods applicable to different varieties of gynecological disorder are introduced briefly as follows:

1. Menstrual Diseases (*Yue Jing Bing*)

For early menstruation categorized as heat, use *Si Wu Tang* (Decoction of Four Ingredients) plus Radix Scutellariae Baicalensis (*Qin*), Rhizoma Coptidis Chinensis (*Lian*), Rhizoma Anemarrhenae (*Zhi*), and Cortex Phellodendri (*Bai*) to clear heat. For delayed menstruation categorized as vacuity cold, use *Si Wu Tang* plus Folium Artemisiae Argyii (*Ai*), Cortex Cinnamomi (*Gui*), Rhizoma Zingiberis (*Jiang*), and Radix Lateralis Praeparatus Aconiti Carmichaeli (*Fu*) to warm cold. For vacuity, add Radix Panacis Ginseng (*Shen*) and Radix Astragali Membranacei (*Qi*). To increase securing and astringing, use Os Draconis (*Long Gu*), Concha Ostreae (*Mu Li*), and carbonized Petiolus Trachycarpi (*Zong Lu Tan*). To increase upbearing and lifting, use Rhizoma Cimicifugae (*Sheng Ma*), Radix Bupleuri (*Chai Hu*), and Folium Nelumbinis Nuciferae (*He Ye*). In conclusion, the discrimination of cold from heat and vacuity from repletion is of utmost therapeutic importance and the administration of medicinals should be flexible in accordance with the signs and symptoms of the individual.

In addition, if menstrual irregularity is the result of other diseases, one should first treat those diseases and, when the disease is eliminated, the menstruation will be automatically regulated. For the same reason, when other ailments are caused by menstrual irregularity, one should first regulate the menstruation. After the menses are regulated, those diseases will automatically be eliminated.

2. Abnormal Vaginal Discharge (*Dai Xia*)

Abnormal vaginal discharge disease is divided into vacuity and repletion. The vacuity pattern mostly pertains to spleen/kidney insufficiency. For treatment it is appropriate to mainly fortify the spleen, dry dampness, and supplement the kidneys. The repletion pattern mostly pertains to damp heat pouring downward. For treatment it is appropriate to mainly clear and disinhibit damp heat.

3. Gestational Diseases (*Ren Shen Bing*)

If some disease is causing restless fetus, one should first treat this disease. When this disease is cured, the fetus will automatically be quieted. If fetal restlessness leads to other diseases, then it is appropriate to first quiet the fetus. When the fetus is quiet, these other diseases will spontaneously be healed. The root of quieting the fetus is nourishing the blood. In general, medicinals used during gestation should be based primarily on nourishing the blood and clearing heat, assisted by fortifying the spleen and rectifying the qi. When the spleen is fortified, the qi and blood are easily engendered. Rectifying the qi leads to normal flow of the qi. The fetus thus also becomes quiet and harmonious. There are three prohibitions during pregnancy. The first prohibition is not to emit sweat. The second prohibition is not to attack and precipitate. The third prohibition is not to disinhibit urination. Sweating leads to perishing of yang and damage of the fluids. Precipitating leads to perishing of yin and damage to the blood. Disinhibition of urination can also damage fluids and humors. However, depending upon the symptoms and pattern of individual patients, one may administer such medicinals when absolutely necessary, but only after careful consideration.

4. Postpartum Diseases (*Chan Hou Bing*)

Postpartum, the proper regulation of lifestyle can reduce the frequency of disease. For instance, if postpartum loss of blood is excessive, the *chong* and *ren* may suffer detriment and damage. Therefore, one should first greatly supplement the qi and blood. However, minor miscellaneous problems present during the puerperium may be left untreated unless they prevent the mother from a speedy recovery. For example, if there is cold congelation and qi stagnation with static blood obstructing internally, it is appropriate to rectify the qi and dispel stasis treating with warming medicinals. In such cases, the methods of dispelling evil and supporting the righteous should be equally emphasized. If postpartum the hundreds of joints are empty and vacuous and the six environmental excesses invade externally, there is repletion in the midst of vacuity. In such cases, it is forbidden to cause great sweating to emit the exterior. Rather, one must take precautions to stop vacuity desertion. If there is damage by food and drink, excessive use of dispersing and conducting is not appropriate. In case of postpartum fever, it is essential to differentiate vacuity and repletion. Vacuity heat should be treated by the sweat warming method. Bedroom taxation may lead to the arising of uterine bleeding and dizziness and fainting. Treatment of this should first greatly supplement the qi and blood. If severe, it should be treated with *Du Shen Tang* (Unaccompanied Ginseng Decoction).

Ancient physicians had the saying, "No insufficiency during gestation; no surplus after delivery", and this is commonly so. However, there can also be insufficiency patterns during gestation, and there may be surplus diseases after delivery. Therefore, one can never be too careful in differentiating the one class of patterns from the other.

5. Breast Diseases (*Ru Bing*)

In the initial stage of breast abscess, one should first mainly scatter the exterior, course the liver, and clear stomach heat. It is also possible to use external treatments. Once pus has formed and begins to weep, treatment should support the interior and evacuate pus. If the skin has broken and the muscles and flesh are not engendered, if pussy water is clear and watery, then treatment should warm and supplement the qi and blood. If lactation is scanty due to the mother's body being debilitated and weak and construction and nourishment (*i.e.*, nutrition) are not good, then it is appropriate to greatly supplement the qi and blood. If the emotions are not smoothly flowing, treatment should soothe the liver and resolve depression at the same time as soothing and smoothing the emotions. Thus lactation will automatically become abundant.

6. Uterine Downward Desertion (*Yin Ting Xia Tuo*)

Uterine downward desertion (*i.e.*, uterine prolapse) is usually due to qi and blood vacuity weakness and loss of restraint of the *dai mai*. Therefore, it is appropriate to supplement the qi, upbear and raise. If there is simultaneously damp heat, it is appropriate to assist this using the methods of transforming dampness and clearing heat.

Chapter Four

Menstrual Diseases (*Yue Jing Bing*)

Menstrual diseases are among the most commonly seen gynecological disorders. Menstrual irregularity affects the general health of the body and is also connected to reproduction. The following is a brief introduction of the disease causes, pathophysiology, diagnosis, treatment, and prevention of menstrual diseases.

Women's menstrual irregularity may manifest various different conditions. In terms of its periodicity, there may be early menstruation, delayed menstruation, or erratic menstruation. In terms of its amount and color, there may be excessive menstruation or astringent, scanty menstruation, and its color may range from purple and black to pale and light. In addition, there is also painful menstruation, uterine bleeding, menstrual movement epistaxis, menstrual movement breast distention and pain, menstrual block (*i.e.*, amenorrhea), and menopausal syndrome. Although varied in form, its causes are invasion by external evils and internal damage due to psycho-emotional causes.

The *Fu Ren Da Quan Liang Fang (A Great, Complete [Collection of] Fine Formulas for Women)* says, "Women's moon water irregularity — there are wind evils invading the uterus and damaging the vessels of the *chong* and *ren*." In clinical practice, one commonly sees that contraction of cold at the time of menstruation leads to the arising of painful menstruation and menstrual block. Damage by cold, malaria-like diseases, and other such diseases can lead to menstrual irregularity or menstrual block. Likewise, psycho-emotional damage is a main cause leading to the arising of menstrual irregularity. Women's emotions are easily stimulated and stirred. If there is excessive worry, thought, resentment, and anger leading to emotional depression, depression may lead to qi binding. Then one's eating and drinking will be affected, leading to a decrease in food and drink. This, in turn, disturbs the source of engenderment and transformation and easily causes the production of menstrual disease. According to Li Dong-yuan, the spleen is the source of engenderment and transformation, while the heart commands the blood of all the channels. If the heart and spleen are level (*i.e.*, calm or healthy) and harmonious, the menstruation arrives at its normally appointed intervals. Internal damage by the seven passions, spleen/stomach vacuity detriment, and heart fire recklessly stirring may all lead to menstrual irregularity. In addition, bedroom affairs excessive beyond limit, sex just prior to the onset of menstruation, eating and drinking chilled, raw things when the period comes, and overtaxation and fatigue during the menstrual period can all also lead to the occurrence of menstrual irregularity.

Diagnosis is based upon inquiry about the menstrual cycle, the color of the menses, the volume of the menses, the consistency of the menses, and upon the discrimination of heat and cold, vacuity and repletion patterns in combination with other generalized signs and symptoms as gathered by the four examinations. Typically, early menstruation is due to heat, while delayed menstruation is due to cold. A dark red colored menstruate is the normal color. A menstruate the color of rice washing water is due to dampness. A pale red menstruate is due to vacuity. A purplish black, dull-colored menstruate with clots is due to cold, while a purplish black, fresh-colored menstruate with clots is due to heat. Menstruation which is excessive in amount is due to replete heat, but if it is scanty and astringent, this is due to vacuity cold. If the substance of the menstruate is thick and pasty and has a foul odor, this is categorized as heat. If it is clear and chilly and without odor, this is categorized as cold.

In terms of treatment principles, emphasis should be on regulating the menstruation so as to treat the root. However, it is also important to treat either before or after other concurrent internal medicine or other diseases. Xiao Sheng-zhai has said:

> Women may either first have disease and then menstrual irregularity, or menstrual irregularity may later cause the engenderment of disease. If first there is disease and then there is menstrual irregularity, first treat the

disease. If there is menstrual irregularity and then there is disease, first regulate the menses. Regulating the menstruation leads to the disease automatically being eliminated.

As it is also said by Wang Meng-ying: "In regulating the menses, it is necessary to first regulate the qi." What this means is that women's menstrual diseases are most often categorized as stagnation of the qi mechanism. Qi is the commander of the blood. Therefore, using medicinals which rectify the qi can never be overstated in the treatment of such cases. However, the principles of treating the branch in acute cases and treating the root in relaxed (*i.e.*, chronic) cases should also be taken into account. If there is profuse uterine bleeding, this is an acute situation and stopping bleeding should be primary. Likewise, in acute painful menstruation, stopping pain is the main thing.

In terms of treatment, principles such as moving the qi and harmonizing the blood, dispelling stasis, diffusing depression, expelling cold, clearing heat, nourishing the blood, and boosting the qi are also frequently applied in using formulas and prescriptions. Specifically, formulas such as *Jia Wei Wu Yao San* (Added Flavors Lindera Powder) and *Yan Hu Suo San* (Corydalis Powder) move the qi. *Jia Wei Si Wu Tang* (Added Flavors Four Materials Decoction) and *Dang Gui Jian Zhong Tang* (Dang Gui Fortify the Center Decoction) harmonize and nourish the blood. *Gui Pi Tang* (Restore the Spleen Decoction) and *Bu Zhong Yi Qi Tang* (Supplement the Center & Boost the Qi Decoction) supplement the qi. *Xiao Yao San* (Rambling Powder) and *Tiao Gan Tang* (Regulate the Liver Decoction) diffuse depression. *Qin Lian Si Wu Tang* (Scutellaria & Coptis Four Materials Decoction) clears heat. *Wen Jing Tang* (Warm the Menses Decoction) or *Wen Jing She Xue Tang* (Warm the Menses & Gather the Blood Decoction) dispel cold. Further explanation of the differentiation of patterns and indications of these various therapies are given below in the following sections.

Important points in the prevention of the onset of menstrual diseases:

1. During the menstruation, bedroom affairs are prohibited. Chilled foods and drinks as well as acrid, hot (*i.e.*, spicy hot) foods are also prohibited.

One should take care not to be invaded by cold and they should protect the warmth of their lower body. Sitting in baths is prohibited and one should take care not to become excessively fatigued.

2. During the menstruation and at other times, one should keep their essence spirit happy and cheerful. If the visceral qi is level and harmonious, then the menstruation will automatically be regulated and normally flowing.

Section One

Early Menstruation (*Yue Jing Xian Qi*)

Menstruation occurring 8-9 days ahead of its expected due date or, in severe cases, menstruation which occurs every half month is referred to as early menstruation. However, if menstruation comes early only once or just 3-5 days early with no other obvious discomfort, this should not be called early menstruation.

Disease Causes, Disease Mechanisms

Blood Heat

Most cases of early menstruation are categorized as heat. This can then be differentiated into replete heat, vacuity heat, depressive heat, and phlegm heat types. Replete heat is mostly caused by constitutional yang exuberance and overeating acrid, hot foods. Vacuity heat mostly results from a constitutional yin vacuity or from enduring disease or blood loss damaging yin. Yin vacuity leads to fire effulgence. Depressive heat is mostly caused by emotional depression transforming into fire. Phlegm heat is commonly due to excessive phlegm in obese persons. Over time, this transforms into fire. Due to the above types of heat forcing the blood to move recklessly, the *chong* and *ren* do not secure, and the menstruation comes before schedule. The *Dan Xi Xin Fa (Dan-xi's Heart Methods)*, says, "Menstrual water not reaching its appointed time and coming is blood heat."

Qi Vacuity /deficiency

Mostly due to undisciplined eating and drinking or taxation and fatigue beyond limit, there is detriment and damage of the spleen qi. The spleen loses its command of the restraint of the blood. Thus qi vacuity is not able to secure and contain the *chong* and *ren*. Therefore there is early menstruation. As Zhang Jing-yue says: "If the pulse and pattern do not have fire and the menses are early, this is heart/spleen vacuity not able to secure and contain the blood."

Disease Patterns

Blood Heat

1. Replete heat: The menstrual blood is excessive in volume and may be dark red in color or purplish and have clots. It may also have a bad odor. There may be paroxysms of lower abdominal pain. There is a red face and oral thirst, desire for chilled drinks, vexatious heat within the heart, low back and knee soreness and weakness, and dry stools. If heat is severe, the eyes are red and there are mouth sores, epistaxis, and other such symptoms. The tongue is red with a yellow coating, and the pulse is slippery and rapid.

2. Vacuity heat: There is early menstruation, but the volume is scanty, and the blood is light and pale. The body is thin and weak, and there is dizziness and vertigo, heart vexation, a dry throat, burning heat in the heart, dry, withered skin, a red tongue with a scant coating, and a fine, rapid pulse.

3. Depressive heat: There is early menstruation and its volume is excessive. There is dizziness, lateral costal pain, chest fullness and oppression, acid eructations and belching, decreased eating and drinking, emotional depression, sluggishness in movement and stirring, frequent sighing, a white tongue coating, and a wiry pulse.

4. Phlegm heat: The volume of menstruation may be either somewhat excessive or not. The body is obese and the face is puffy and yellow. There

29

is head distention like a band, the limbs are heavy, and there is vertigo, chest oppression, excessive phlegm, desire to vomit, possible loose stools, abdominal distention, and chronic abnormal vaginal discharge. The tongue coating is white and slimy or slightly yellow. The pulse is slippery and rapid.

Qi Vacuity

There is early menstruation which is pale in color and excessive in volume. There is essence spirit fatigue, dizziness and vertigo, heart palpitations, racing heart, a cold body and fear of chill, a forceless voice, no flavor of food and drink or no thought for food or drink, a pale red, thin, moist tongue or a vacuous red, fat and enlarged tongue, and a soft, weak, forceless pulse image.

Treatment

Hot Blood

1. Replete Heat: One should clear heat from the blood aspect. The formula to use is Master Fu's (*i.e.* Fu Qing-zhu's) *Qing Jing San* (Clear the Menses Powder) or *Qin Lian Su Wu Tang* (Scutellaria & Coptis Four Materials Decoction). If there is simultaneous abdominal pain, one can add Fructus Meliae Toosendan (*Chuan Lian Zi*) and Rhizoma Corydalis Yanhusuo (*Yan Hu Suo*).

2. Vacuity Heat: One should nourish yin and clear heat. The formula to use is *Liang Di Tang* (Two *Di* Decoction).

3. Depressive Heat: One should sooth and resolve liver/spleen depression. The formula to use is *Jia Wei Xiao Yao San* (Added Flavors Rambling Powder). If due to excessive angry qi resulting in depressive heat, then one may use *Yi Guan Jian Jia Jian* (One Link Decoction with Additions & Subtractions).

4. Phlegm Heat: One should eliminate dampness, transform phlegm, and clear heat. According to the *Dan Xi Xin Fa (Dan-xi's Heart Methods)*, pills can be made from Rhizoma Gastrodiae Elatae (*Tian Ma*), Rhizoma Atractylodis Macrocephalae (*Bai Zhu*), Rhizoma Atractylodis (*Cang Zhu*), Rhizoma Coptidis Chinensis (*Huang Lian*), Rhizoma Cyperi Rotundi (*Xiang Fu*), and Radix Ligustici Wallichii (*Chuan Xiong*).

Qi Vacuity

One should supplement the qi and contain the blood. The formula to use is *Gui Pi Tang* (Restore the Spleen Decoction), *Bu Zhong Yi Qi Tang Jia Jian* (Supplement the Center & Boost the Qi Decoction with Additions & Subtractions), or *Si Wu Tang* (Four Materials Decoction) plus Radix Codonopsis Pilosulae (*Dang Shen*), Rhizoma Atractylodis Macrocephalae (*Bai Zhu*), Radix Astragali Membranacei (*Huang Qi*), Fructus Schizandrae Chinensis (*Wu Wei Zi*), and Pericarpium Citri Reticulatae (*Chen Pi*).

Explanation

1. The patient's age and general health has a bearing on the diagnosis and treatment of this disorder. For example, if early menstruation happens in a woman of robust health with abdominal pain followed by dark red discharge or by profuse, purple menstrual discharge, this often suggests heat and repletion. Nevertheless, if early menstruation develops in an older woman who likes pressure on her abdomen after her period has begun with scant volume and light color and who at the same time suffers from fatigue and poor appetite, the vacuous nature of this disorder can then be established.

2. If the excessive menstrual discharge remains unchecked, those with hot blood can be treated with the same prescriptions given above but with the addition of carbonized Radix Scutellariae Baicalensis (*Huang Qin*), carbonized Cacumen Biotae Orientalis (*Ce Bai Ye*), and carbonized Radix Sanguisorbae (*Di Yu*). The aim of these additional ingredients is to aid in clearing heat and stop the bleeding. On the other hand, for those with qi

31

vacuity, Crinis Carbonisatus (*Xue Yu Tan*), carbonized Petiolus Trachycarpi (*Zong Lu Tan*), and Concha Ostreae (*Mu Li*) may be added to secure, contain, and stop bleeding.

Appended Formulas

1. *Qing Jing San* (from *Fu Qing Zhu Nu Ke [Fu Qing-zhu's Gynecology]*): Cortex Radicis Moutan (*Dan Pi*), stir-fried Rhizoma Atractylodis Macrocephalae (*Bai Zhu*), prepared Radix Rehmanniae (*Shu Di*), Cortex Radicis Lycii Chinensis (*Di Gu Pi*), Sclerotium Poriae Cocos (*Fu Ling*), Cortex Phellodendri (*Huang Bai*), Herba Artemisiae Apiaceae (*Qing Hao*)

2. *Qin Lian Si Wu Tang* (from *Shen Shi Zun Sheng Shu [Master Shen's Writings on Respecting Life]*): Radix Angelicae Sinensis (*Dang Gui*), Radix Ligustici Wallichii (*Chuan Xiong*), Radix Albus Paeoniae Lactiflorae (*Bai Shao*), Radix Rehmanniae (*Di Huang*), Radix Scutellariae Baicalensis (*Huang Qin*), Rhizoma Coptidis Chinensis (*Huang Lian*)

3. *Liang Di Tang* (from *Fu Qing Zhu Nu Ke [Fu Qing-zhu's Gynecology]*): Uncooked Radix Rehmanniae (*Da Sheng Di*), Cortex Radicis Lycii Chinensis (*Di Gu Pi*), Radix Scrophulariae Ningpoensis (*Xuan Shen*), Radix Albus Paeoniae Lactiflorae (*Bai Shao*), Tuber Ophiopogonis Japonicae (*Mai Dong*), Gelatinum Corii Asini (*E Jiao*)

4. *Jia Wei Xiao Yao San:* Radix Angelicae Sinensis (*Dang Gui*), Radix Albus Paeoniae Lactiflorae (*Bai Shao*), Radix Bupleuri (*Chai Hu*), Sclerotium Poriae Cocos (*Fu Ling*), Radix Glycyrrhizae (*Gan Cao*), Rhizoma Atractylodis Macrocephalae (*Bai Zhu*), Herba Menthae Haplocalysis (*Bo He*), Rhizoma Cyperi Rotundi (*Xiang Fu*), Herba Lycopi Lucidi (*Ze Lan*), uncooked Radix Rehmanniae (*Sheng Di*), Tuber Curcumae (*Yu Jin*), Fructus Gardeniae Jasminoidis (*Zhi Zi*), Radix Scutellariae Baicalensis (*Huang Qin*)

5. *Yi Guan Jian* (Wei Zhi-xiu's formula)*:* Uncooked Radix Rehmanniae (*Sheng Di*), Radix Angelicae Sinensis (*Dang Gui*), Fructus Lycii Chinensis (*Gou Qi Zi*), Radix Glehniae Littoralis (*Sha Shen*), Tuber Ophiopogonis

Japonicae (*Mai Dong*), stir-fried Fructus Meliae Toosendan (*Chuan Lian Zi*)

6. *Gui Pi Tang* (from *Ji Sheng Fang [Formulas for the Aid of the Living]*): Radix Codonopsis Pilosulae (*Dang Shen*), mix-fried Radix Astragali Membranacei (*Huang Qi*), Radix Angelicae Sinensis (*Dang Gui*), Rhizoma Atractylodis Macrocephalae (*Bai Zhu*), mix-fried Radix Glycyrrhizae (*Zhi Gan Cao*), Radix Saussureae Seu Vladimiriae (*Mu Xiang*), Semen Zizyphi Spinosae (*Suan Zao Ren*), Radix Polygalae Tenuifoliae (*Yuan Zhi*), Sclerotium Poriae Cocos (*Fu Ling*), Arillus Euphoriae Longanae (*Long Yan Rou*), uncooked Rhizoma Zingiberis (*Sheng Jiang*), Fructus Zizyphi Jujubae (*Da Zao*)

7. *Bu Zhong Yi Qi Tang* (from *Pi Wei Lun [Treatise on the Spleen & Stomach]*): Radix Astragali Membranacei (*Huang Qi*), Rhizoma Atractylodis Macrocephalae (*Bai Zhu*), Radix Codonopsis Pilosulae (*Dang Shen*), Pericarpium Citri Reticulatae (*Chen Pi*), Rhizoma Cimicifugae (*Sheng Ma*), Radix Bupleuri (*Chai Hu*), Radix Angelicae Sinensis (*Dang Gui*), mix-fried Radix Glycyrrhizae (*Zhi Gan Cao*), Fructus Zizyphi Jujubae (*Da Zao*), dry Rhizoma Zingiberis (*Gan Jiang*).

8. *Si Wu Tang* (from the *Tai Ping Hui Min He Ji Ju Fang [Tai Ping Imperial Grace Formulary]*): Prepared Radix Rehmanniae (*Shu Di*), Radix Angelicae Sinensis (*Dang Gui*), Radix Ligustici Wallichii (*Chuan Xiong*), Radix Albus Paeoniae Lactiflorae (*Bai Shao*)

Section Two

Delayed Menstruation (*Yue Jing Hou Qi*)

If menstruation commonly occurs at least 7-8 or even more than 10 days later than its expected due date, this is called delayed menstruation, late menstruation, or slow menstruation. If it occurs only 3-5 days late, is not accompanied by any other symptoms, and only happens one time, this should not be called delayed menstruation.

Disease Causes, Disease Mechanisms

The causes of this disease are divided into the four types of: blood vacuity, blood cold, qi stagnation, and phlegm obstruction.

Blood Vacuity

This is mostly due to blood loss or the aftermath of enduring disease when the constructive and blood are insufficient and the sea of blood is empty and vacuous. Thus it is not able to fill itself and become exuberant in time and to then descend. Therefore it is behind schedule. Zhu Dan-xi says, "Late periods are the result of blood vacuity."

Blood Cold

This is due to yang qi insufficiency and the engenderment of cold internally. Yin cold may also enter from outside and engender chill which damages internally. Thus the blood becomes cold and congealed. The blood vessels are not smoothly flowing and hence the period is late.

Qi Stagnation

This is mostly due to emotional depression leading to blood movement not being smooth. The *chong* and *ren* thus suffer obstruction. If severe, this results in stasis binding. The *Yi Zong Jin Jian (Golden Mirror of Ancestral Medicine)* says:

> Menstrual movement behind schedule, if colored purple and the blood is
> scant and if there is abdominal distention and pain, this is categorized as
> qi repletion and blood stasis and stagnation.

Phlegm Obstruction

This is commonly due, in obese persons, to excessive phlegm turbidity which obstructs and stagnates in the *chong* and *ren*. Thus the menstruation is not able to respond in a timely manner and descend.

Disease Patterns

Blood Vacuity

The menstruation is behind schedule. Its color is pale and volume is scanty. The facial complexion is somber white and there are heart palpitations, scanty sleep, dizziness, tinnitus, possible tidal fever in the afternoon, lack of moisture of the skin, dry stools, and a vacuous, fine or fine, rapid pulse.

Blood Cold

The menstrual water is behind schedule. Its color is dark and not fresh or is purplish black. Its amount is scanty. There is lower abdominal aching and pain, aversion to cold and desire for warmth, a somber white facial complexion, chilling of the four limbs, possible poor appetite, low back and lower leg soreness and weakness, a pale tongue with a thin coating, and a deep, tight pulse.

Qi Stagnation

The menstruation is late. Its amount is scanty, its color is dark, and it contains clots. There is lower abdominal distention and pain, epigastric, lateral costal, and breast distention, a thin tongue coating, and a wiry pulse.

Phlegm Obstruction

The menstrual water is behind schedule. If severe, it may only come once in several months. The color of the menstruation is pale and its volume is scanty. There is chronic abnormal vaginal discharge, chest oppression, epigastric distention, excessive phlegm, essence spirit fatigue, a vacuous, puffy facial complexion, heavy limbs, dizziness, heart palpitations, and shortness of breath. The tongue has a white, slimy coating, and the pulse is wiry and slippery.

35

Treatment

Blood Vacuity

One should nourish the blood and boost the qi. The formulas to use are *Ren Shen Yang Rong Tang* (Ginseng Nourish the Constructive Decoction) and *Ren Shen Zi Xue Tang* (Ginseng Enrich the Blood Decoction). If yin vacuity pattern appears, one may use *Ren Shen Gu Ben Wan* (Ginseng Secure the Root Decoction).

Blood Cold

One should warm the channels and scatter cold, move the qi and harmonize the stomach. The formula to use is *Wen Jing Tang* (Warm the Menses Decoction) or *Wu Yao San* (Lindera Powder) with added flavors, such as Cortex Eucommiae Ulmoidis (*Du Zhong*) and Radix Dipsaci (*Chuan Duan*) in case of low back soreness. Another alternative prescription is *Si Wu Tang* (Four Materials Decoction) with the addition of Folium Artemisiae Argyii (*Ai Ye*), Rhizoma Cyperi Rotundi (*Xiang Fu*), Fructus Evodiae Rutecarpae (*Wu Zhu Yu*), and Ramulus Cinnamomi (*Gui Zhi*).

Qi Stagnation

Course the liver and rectify the qi, quicken the blood and regulate menstruation. The formula to use is *Xiao Yao San* (Rambling Powder) or *Chai Hu Si Wu Tang* (Bupleurum Four Materials Decoction) plus Rhizoma Cyperi Rotundi (*Xiang Fu*), Tuber Curcumae (*Yu Jin*), Radix Salviae Miltiorrhizae (*Dan Shen*), Fructus Citri Sacrodactylis (*Fo Shou*), and Flos Pruni Mume (*Lu O Mei*).

Phlegm Obstruction

Fortify the spleen and transform phlegm. The formula to use is *Xiang Sha Liu Jun Zi Tang* (Saussurea & Amomum Six Gentlemen Decoction). Or, to transform phlegm and nourish the blood, the formula to use is *Xiong Gui Er Chen Tang* (Ligusticum & Dang Gui Two Aged [Ingredients]

Decoction) or *Gui Shao Liu Jun Zi Tang* (Dang Gui & Peony Six Gentlemen Decoction).

Explanation

1. In case of delayed menstruation, it is important to analyze the amount of menstruation, its color, viscosity, and whether there is abdominal pain. Typically, if there is delayed menstruation, its color purple, its volume scanty, and there is simultaneous abdominal pain, by far this is mostly due to cold congelation, qi stagnation, or blood stasis. If its color is pale, its amount is scanty, and there is no abdominal pain, by far this is mostly blood vacuity or phlegm obstruction.

2. In case of delayed menstruation, it is essential to make sure that there is no pregnancy or fetal leakage. One should take care in their diagnosis, pulse, and patterns and one should also take care in using medicinals for moving the qi and breaking the blood.

3. In blood vacuity delayed menstruation, usually the heart and lungs have suffered detriment. If this remains untreated for a long time, blood withering will result in menstrual block. Typically, such patients will have symptoms of vacuity heat accompanied by a fine, rapid pulse. Treatment should mainly nourish the blood and enrich yin. Acrid, hot medicinals which consume yin fluids are prohibited.

Appended Formulas

1. *Ren Shen Yang Rong Tang* (from *Tai Ping Hui Min He Ji Ju Fang [Tai Ping Imperial Grace Formulary])*: Radix Panacis Ginseng (*Ren Shen*), Pericarpium Citri Reticulatae (*Chen Pi*), mix-fried Radix Astragali Membranacei (*Huang Qi*), Cortex Cinnamomi (*Rou Gui*), scorched Rhizoma Atractylodis Macrocephalae (*Bai Zhu*), mix-fried Radix Glycyrrhizae (*Zhi Gan Cao*), wine stir-fried Radix Albus Paeoniae Lactiflorae (*Bai Shao*), prepared Radix Rehmanniae (*Shu Di*), Fructus Schizandrae Chinensis (*Wu Wei Zi*), Sclerotium Poriae Cocos (*Fu Ling*), Radix Polygalae Tenuifoliae (*Yuan Zhi*), Radix Angelicae Sinensis (*Dang Gui*)

2. *Ren Shen Zi Xue Tang* (from *Chan Bao Bai Wen [One Hundred Questions about Birthing]*): Radix Panacis Ginseng (*Ren Shen*), Radix Dioscoreae Oppositae (*Shan Yao*), Sclerotium Poriae Cocos (*Fu Ling*), Radix Ligustici Wallichii (*Chuan Xiong*), wine stir-fried Radix Albus Paeoniae Lactiflorae (*Bai Shao*), prepared Radix Rehmanniae (*Shu Di*), Radix Angelicae Sinensis (*Dang Gui*)

3. *Ren Shen Gu Ben Wan* (from *Ye Shi Nu Ke [Master Ye's Gynecology]*): Radix Panacis Ginseng (*Ren Shen*), uncooked Radix Rehmanniae (*Sheng Di*), prepared Radix Rehmanniae (*Shu Di*), Tuber Asparagi Cochinensis (*Tian Dong*), and Tuber Ophiopogonis Japonicae (*Mai Dong*).

4. *Wu Yao San Jia Wei* (from *Yi Zong Jin Jian [Golden Mirror of Ancestral Medicine]*): Radix Linderae Strychnifoliae (*Wu Yao*), Rhizoma Cyperi Rotundi (*Xiang Fu*), Sclerotium Poriae Cocos (*Fu Ling*), Pericarpium Citri Reticulatae (*Chen Pi*), Fructus Crataegi (*Shan Zha*), Radix Angelicae Sinensis (*Dang Gui*), stir-fried Radix Albus Paeoniae Lactiflorae (*Bai Shao*), processed Rhizoma Corydalis Yanhusuo (*Yan Hu Suo*), Ramulus Cinnamomi (*Gui Zhi*)

5. *Wen Jing Tang* (from *Jin Gui Yao Lue [Essentials from the Golden Cabinet]*):Radix Angelicae Sinensis (*Dang Gui*), Radix Ligustici Wallichii (*Chuan Xiong*), Radix Panacis Ginseng (*Ren Shen*), Gelatinum Corii Asini (*E Jiao*), Radix Glycyrrhizae (*Gan Cao*), Cortex Cinnamomi (*Rou Gui*), stir-fried Radix Albus Paeoniae Lactiflorae (*Bai Shao*), Fructus Evodiae Rutecarpae (*Wu Zhu Yu*), Cortex Radicis Moutan (*Dan Pi*), Tuber Ophiopogonis Japonicae (*Mai Dong*), Rhizoma Pinelliae Ternatae (*Ban Xia*), uncooked Rhizoma Zingiberis (*Sheng Jiang*)

6. *Xiao Yao San* (from *Tai Ping Hui Min He Ji Ju Fang [Tai Ping Imperial Grace Formulary]*): Radix Angelicae Sinensis (*Dang Gui*), stir-fried Radix Albus Paeoniae Lactiflorae (*Bai Shao*), Sclerotium Poriae Cocos (*Fu Ling*), mix-fried Radix Glycyrrhizae (*Zhi Gan Cao*), Radix Bupleuri (*Chai Hu*), Herba Menthae Haplocalycis (*Bo He*), blast-fried Rhizoma Zingiberis (*Pao Jiang*), Rhizoma Atractylodis Macrocephalae (*Bai Zhu*)

7. *Chai Hu Si Wu Tang:* Uncooked Radix Rehmanniae (*Sheng Di*), Radix Ligustici Wallichii (*Chuan Xiong*), Radix Albus Paeoniae Lactiflorae (*Bai Shao*), Radix Angelicae Sinensis (*Dang Gui*), Radix Bupleuri (*Chai Hu*)

8. *Xiang Sha Liu Jun Zi Tang:* Radix Codonopsis Pilosulae (*Dang Shen*), Sclerotium Poriae Cocos (*Fu Ling*), Rhizoma Atractylodis Macrocephalae (*Bai Zhu*), mix-fried Radix Glycyrrhizae (*Zhi Gan Cao*), Pericarpium Citri Reticulatae (*Chen Pi*), Rhizoma Pinelliae Ternatae (*Ban Xia*), Radix Saussureae Seu Vladimiriae, Fructus Amomi (*Sha Ren*)

9. *Xiong Gui Er Chen Tang* (from *Zheng Zhi Zhun Sheng [Patterns & Treatments Norms & Criteria]*): Radix Ligustici Wallichii (*Chuan Xiong*), Radix Angelicae Sinensis (*Dang Gui*), Pericarpium Citri Reticulatae (*Chen Pi*), Rhizoma Pinelliae Ternatae (*Ban Xia*), Sclerotium Poriae Cocos (*Fu Ling*), mix-fried Radix Glycyrrhizae (*Zhi Gan Cao*)

10. *Gui Shao Liu Jun Zi Tang:* Radix Angelicae Sinensis (*Dang Gui*), wine stir-fried Radix Albus Paeoniae Lactiflorae (*Bai Shao*), Radix Codonopsis Pilosulae (*Dang Shen*), stir-fried Rhizoma Atractylodis Macrocephalae (*Bai Zhu*), Sclerotium Poriae Cocos (*Fu Ling*), mix-fried Radix Glycyrrhizae (*Zhi Gan Cao*)

Section Three

Early, Late, Erratic Menstruation (*Yue Jing Qian Hou Wu Ding Qi*)

If the menstruation constantly comes sometimes early, sometimes late, and its periodicity is chaotic and confused, this is called early, late, erratic menstruation. It is also called transgressing its schedule menstruation.

Disease Causes, Disease Mechanisms

The onset of this disease is mainly due to qi and blood irregularity. Thus the function of the *chong* and *ren* is chaotic and confused and there is loss of normalcy in the sea of blood's storing and spillage. The cause of this qi and blood irregularity and chaos and confusion in the function of the *chong* and *ren* is due to liver depression, kidney vacuity, and spleen vacuity. Angry qi damages the liver. The liver qi thus becomes depressed and stagnant. The qi mechanism counterflows and becomes chaotic. Or it is possible that liver qi is insufficient due to undisciplined bedroom affairs, and excessive reproduction. Thus the *chong* and *ren* suffer detriment and damage. This also can cause the menstruation to be chaotic. In addition, if the spleen qi is debilitated and weak, water and grain cannot be made into the constructive and blood. This also may lead to the menstruation being early, late, and erratic. As it is said in the *Ye Tian Shi Nu Ke (Ye Tian-shi's Gynecology)*:

> Menstruation, sometimes early, sometimes late — this is due to spleen earth not being victorious. There is no thought for food or drink. This causes blood vacuity and thus the menstrual waters are late. Or some months, eating and drinking are excessive. Thus the menstruation comes early.

Disease Patterns

Kidney Vacuity

The menstruation is sometimes early and sometimes late. Its color is a fresh red and simultaneously there is white vaginal discharge. In the wake of menstruation, there is lower and upper back soreness and pain and heavy pain in the lower abdomen. There is also dizziness, tinnitus, dreams of intercourse at night, and frequent, numerous urination. The tongue is pale with a thin coating, and the pulse is deep, weak, and fine.

Liver Depression

The menstruation comes early, late, and erratically. Its initial movement is not smooth. Its amount may be either excessive or scanty. There is lower abdominal distention and pain, chest and lateral costal or breast distention and pain, belching, poor appetite, and possibly a bitter taste in the mouth. The tongue coating is thin and white, and the pulse is wiry.

Spleen Vacuity

The menstruation comes either early or late. Its amount is excessive or dribbling and dripping without stop. Its color is pale red. There is shortness of breath, lack of strength, dizziness, heart palpitations, devitalized appetite, and loose stools. The tongue coating is white and slimy, and the pulse is vacuous, relaxed (*i.e.*, retarded), and forceless.

Treatment

Kidney Vacuity

One should enrich yin and supplement the kidneys, regulate and boost the *chong* and *ren*. The formulas to use are *Zi Yin Ba Wei Wan* (Enrich Yin Eight Flavors Pills) and *Gu Yin Jian* (Secure Yin Decoction).

Liver Depression

One should soothe the liver and resolve depression. The formula to use is *Xiao Yao San* minus Herba Menthae Haplocalycis (*Bo He*) and blast-fried Rhizoma Zingiberis (*Pao Jiang*) and plus Tuber Curcumae (*Yu Jin*), Radix Ligustici Wallichii (*Chuan Xiong*), Rhizoma Cyperi Rotundi (*Xiang Fu*), Fructus Meliae Toosendan (*Chuan Lian Zi*), and Fructus Citri Sacrodactylis (*Fo Shou Pian*).

Spleen Vacuity

One should fortify the spleen and warm the stomach. The formula to use is *Wen Wei Yin* (Warm the Stomach Drink). If there are loose stools, remove the Radix Angelicae Sinensis (*Dang Gui*).

Explanation

1. This disease may be due to excessive bedroom affairs. The *chong* and *ren* thus suffer detriment which leads to kidney qi vacuity and deficiency. In addition, pregnancy during early adolescence may also easily result in this disease. Correspondingly, one should discipline and regulate their bedroom affairs and not become pregnant too young in life. Thus this disease will be prevented.

2. If this disease endures for a long time, not only will it affect conception and reproduction, it will lead to qi and blood vanquishing and chaos. This then easily leads to the arising of uterine bleeding patterns. Therefore, one should not overlook its treatment.

3. A number of patients are clinically encountered with irregular menstruation who also complain of low back and knee soreness and weakness apart from all the liver qi depression symptoms. Such patients have liver/kidney qi depression. In clinical practice, Fu Qing-zhu's *Ding Jing Tang* (Stabilize the Menses Decoction) gets good results in such cases. This formula is able to soothe liver/kidney depression and also supplement liver/kidney essence. Thus *yi* and *gui* (*i.e.*, wood and water) are both treated, the qi is soothed and the essence is freed, the movement of the menses automatically becomes stable.

Appended Formulas

1. *Zi Yin Ba Wei Wan:* Prepared Radix Rehmanniae (*Shu Di*), Radix Dioscoreae Oppositae (*Shan Yao*), Fructus Corni Officinalis (*Shan Zhu Yu*), Cortex Radicis Moutan (*Dan Pi*), Rhizoma Alismatis (*Ze Xie*), Sclerotium Poriae Cocos (*Fu Ling*), saltwater stir-fried Cortex Phellodendri (*Huang Bai*), saltwater stir-fried Rhizoma Anemarrhenae (*Zhi Mu*)

2. *Gu Yin Jian* (from *Jing Yue Quan Shu [Jing-yue's Complete Writings]*): Radix Panacis Ginseng (*Ren Shen*), Radix Dioscoreae Oppositae (*Shan Yao*), prepared Radix Rehmanniae (*Shu Di*), Fructus Corni Officinalis

(*Shan Zhu Yu*), Radix Polygalae Tenuifoliae (*Yuan Zhi*), mix-fried Radix Glycyrrhizae (*Zhi Gan Cao*), Fructus Schizandrae Chinensis (*Wu Wei Zi*), Semen Cuscutae (*Tu Si Zi*)

3. *Xiao Yao San:* See Section Two, same chapter.

4. *Wen Wei Yin* (from *Jing Yue Quan Shu [Jing-yue's Complete Writings]*): Radix Panacis Ginseng (*Ren Shen*), stir-fried Rhizoma Atractylodis Macrocephalae (*Bai Zhu*), Semen Dolichoris Lablabis (*Bian Dou*), Pericarpium Citri Reticulatae (*Chen Pi*), uncooked Rhizoma Zingiberis (*Sheng Jiang*), mix-fried Radix Glycyrrhizae (*Zhi Gan Cao*), Radix Angelicae Sinensis (*Dang Gui*)

5. *Ding Jing Tang* (from *Fu Qing Zhu Nu Ke [Fu Qing-zhu's Gynecology]*): Semen Cuscutae (*Tu Si Zi*), Radix Albus Paeoniae Lactiflorae (*Bai Shao*), Radix Angelicae Sinensis (*Dang Gui*), prepared Radix Rehmanniae (*Shu Di*), Radix Dioscoreae Oppositae (*Shan Yao*), Sclerotium Poriae Cocos (*Fu Ling*), Herba Seu Flos Schizonepetae Tenuifoliae (*Jing Jie*), Radix Bupleuri (*Chai Hu*)

Section Four

Excessive Menstruation (*Yue Jing Guo Duo*)

If the menstrual period is normal but the amount of menstruation is obviously much more than normal or if the menstruation comes and lasts for many days and is excessive, this is called excessive menstruation.

Disease Causes, Disease Mechanisms

Due to constitutional yang exuberance or excessive eating of acrid, peppery foods, the blood aspect brews heat which forces the blood to move recklessly. The *Nei Jing (Inner Classic)* says, "If heaven has summerheat

43

and earth has heat, the menstrual water may boil and spill over." This is often the case. It is also possible that having bedroom affairs during the menstrual period damages and causes detriment to the *chong* and *ren* and blood network vessels. Also, heart/spleen qi vacuity and taxation and fatigue beyond limit may cause the central qi to fall downward. The qi thus loses its command over containing and grasping. Therefore, this condition is divided into the three types of: blood heat, *chong* and *ren* suffering detriment, and qi vacuity not containing.

Disease Patterns

Blood Heat

Menstruation comes ahead schedule and the volume of the menstruation is excessive. The color of the menses is fresh red or purplish. There is oral thirst, desire to drink, heart vexation, a red face, difficulty sleeping at night, yellow urine, and constipation. The tongue is red with a yellow coating. The pulse is slippery and rapid.

Detriment of the *Chong & Ren*

There is either excessive menstruation or prolonged duration. There is also abdominal pain which likes pressure, soreness of the four extremities, dizziness, blurred vision, lack of flavor of food and drink, a pale tongue with a white coating, and a wiry, fine, forceless pulse.

Qi Vacuity Not Containing

There is either excessive menstruation or prolonged menstruation accompanied by bodily vacuity weakness, a sallow yellow facial complexion, no fragrance to food or drink, a thin, white tongue coating, and a fine, weak pulse.

Treatment

Blood Heat

One should clear heat and foster yin, enrich the liver and nourish the blood. The formula to use is *Dang Gui Yin* (Dang Gui Drink). If uterine bleeding does not stop for many days, add Gelatinum Corii Asini (*E Jiao*), stir-fried Fructus Gardeniae Jasminoidis (*Zhi Zi*), carbonized Radix Sanguisorbae (*Di Yu*), carbonized Herba Seu Flos Schizonepetae Tenuifoliae (*Jing Jie*), Radix Glycyrrhizae (*Gan Cao*), and juice of Rhizoma Phragmitis Communis (*Lu Gen*).

Detriment of the *Chong* and *Ren*

One should supplement the qi and nourish the blood, regulate and rectify the *chong* and *ren*. The formula to use is *Jiao Ai Tang* (Donkey Skin Glue & Mugwort Decoction). If precipitation of blood is excessive, one may add Radix Sanguisorbae (*Di Yu*) and Radix Astragali Membranacei (*Huang Qi*). Or one can use *Bu Zhong Xiong Gui Tang* (Supplement the Center Ligusticum & Dang Gui Decoction).

Qi Vacuity Not Containing

One should supplement the qi and contain the blood. The formula to use is *Gui Pi Tang* (Restore the Spleen Decoction). Or one can use *Jiao Ai Ba Zhen Tang* (Donkey Skin Glue & Mugwort Eight Pearls Decoction).

Explanation

1. In most cases, excessive menstruation and early menstruation are categorized as heat. Excessive menstruation and menstruation which continues on too long and does not stop is mostly categorized as qi vacuity.

2. If women who are past 7x7 years of age whose *tian gui* has already ceased experience the coming of their period which is excessive in amount

but unaccompanied by other signs and symptoms, this is due to their *tian gui*'s cessation being reversed. It is not categorized as a disease.

3. Excessive menstruation is bound to cause yin blood insufficiency. This may manifest as dizziness, heart palpitations, shortness of breath, lack of strength of the four limbs, a somber white facial complexion, etc. If severe, this is liable to transform into massive metrorrhagia unless the treatment is given before it is too late.

Appended Formulas

1. *Dang Gui Yin* (from *Ji Yin Gang Mu [Detailed Outline of Yin, i.e., Women]*): Stir-fried Radix Angelicae Sinensis (*Dang Gui*), Radix Ligustici Wallichii (*Chuan Xiong*), Radix Albus Paeoniae Lactiflorae (*Bai Shao*), prepared Radix Rehmanniae (*Shu Di*), Rhizoma Atractylodis Macrocephalae (*Bai Zhu*), Radix Scutellariae Baicalensis (*Huang Qin*)

2. *Jiao Ai Tang* (from *Jin Gui Yao Lue [Essentials from the Golden Cabinet]*): Prepared Radix Rehmanniae (*Shu Di*), Radix Albus Paeoniae Lactiflorae (*Bai Shao*), Radix Angelicae Sinensis (*Dang Gui*), Folium Artemisiae Argyii (*Ai Ye*), Gelatinum Corii Asini (*E Jiao*), Radix Ligustici Wallichii (*Chuan Xiong*), mix-fried Radix Glycyrrhizae (*Zhi Gan Cao*)

3. *Bu Zhong Xiong Gui Tang* (from *Zheng Zhi Zhun Sheng [Patterns & Treatments Norms & Criteria]*): Radix Angelicae Sinensis (*Dang Gui*), dry Rhizoma Zingiberis (*Gan Jiang*), Radix Ligustici Wallichii (*Chuan Xiong*), prepared Radix Rehmanniae (*Shu Di*), mix-fried Radix Astragali Membranacei (*Huang Qi*), Radix Panacis Ginseng (*Ren Shen*), Cortex Eucommiae Ulmoidis (*Du Zhong*), stir-fried Fructus Evodiae Rutecarpae (*Wu Zhu Tu*), mix-fried Radix Glycyrrhizae (*Zhi Gan Cao*)

4. *Gui Pi Tang:* See Section One, same chapter.

5. *Jiao Ai Ba Zhen Tang:* Radix Codonopsis Pilosulae (*Dang Shen*), Rhizoma Atractylodis Macrocephalae (*Bai Zhu*), Sclerotium Poriae Cocos (*Fu Ling*), mix-fried Radix Glycyrrhizae (*Zhi Gan Cao*), prepared Radix

Rehmanniae (*Shu Di*), Radix Albus Paeoniae Lactiflorae (*Bai Shao*), Radix Angelicae Sinensis (*Dang Gui*), Radix Ligustici Wallichii (*Chuan Xiong*), Gelatinum Corii Asini (*E Jiao*), Folium Artemisiae Argyii (*Ai Ye*)

Section Five

Scanty Menstruation (*Yue Jing Guo Shao*)

If the menstrual period is normal but the amount of menstruation is obviously decreased or is only a few drops, this is called scanty menstruation. This disease commonly becomes menstrual block (*i.e.*, amenorrhea). The menstruation ceases and does not resume. It indicates that the *tian gui* is just about to reach the end of its course, in which case, women will experience a progressively decreasing menstrual flow.

Disease Causes, Disease Mechanisms

Scanty menstruation can be divided into the two types of vacuity and repletion.

The vacuity pattern can be further divided into the two types of blood vacuity and kidney vacuity. Blood vacuity is mostly due to enduring disease or may be seen in the aftermath of a very great disease in which case there is yin blood insufficiency. It may also be due to eating and drinking and taxation and fatigue damaging the spleen. Thus the source of engenderment and transformation is insufficient. This then results in the amount of blood moving being scanty. Kidney vacuity is mostly due to natural endowment kidney qi insufficiency or to excessive births and bedroom taxation. The *chong* and *ren* are taxed and damaged and the sea of blood is not exuberant. Hence this condition occurs.

Repletion patterns can be divided into the two types of blood stasis and phlegm dampness. Blood stasis is mostly due to qi stagnation or cold evils causing obstruction. Therefore, the movement of the blood is not smooth.

47

Phlegm dampness is mostly due to spleen yang loss of transportation. Dampness thus gathers and turns into phlegm. This stagnates in the *chong* and *ren* and therefore the menstrual movement is scanty in amount.

Disease Patterns

Blood Vacuity

The amount of the menstrual water is scanty and its color is pale or its is reduced to only a few drops. There is insidious pain in the lower abdomen or pain which likes pressures, dizziness, heart palpitations, a lusterless facial complexion, a pale tongue with a thin, white coating, and a fine, weak pulse.

Kidney Vacuity

When the menses come, their amount is scant and color is pale red or fresh red. There is low back and knee soreness and weakness, aching and pain in the heels or soles of the feet, dizziness, tinnitus, and going to sleep may be difficult. The tongue is pale with scanty fluids, and the pulse is deep and fine.

Blood Stasis

The amount of the menses is astringent and scanty. Their color is darkish purple and they contain clots. There is lower abdominal distention and pain which refuses pressure or there is qi stagnation with the appearance of lateral costal distention and pain. The tongue is purple and dark or may have static spots. The pulse is deep and choppy or wiry.

Phlegm Dampness

The menstrual movement is scanty in volume. There is bodily fatigue and exhaustion. The feet and lower legs are sore and weak. There is chest and epigastric fullness and oppression and excessive phlegm turbidity. The tongue coating is white and glossy or thick and slimy. The pulse is wiry and slippery or deep and fine.

Treatment

Blood Vacuity

One should first supplement the blood, assisted by boosting the qi. If the qi and blood are effulgent and exuberant, the menstrual blood will automatically be sufficient. The formula to use is *Si Wu Tang* (Four Materials Decoction) plus Radix Pseudostellariae (*Tai Zi Shen*), Fructus Lycii Chinensis (*Gou Qi Zi*), Radix Salviae Miltiorrhizae (*Dan Shen*), Gelatinum Corii Asini (*E Jiao*), and Rhizoma Atractylodis Macrocephalae (*Bai Zhu*). Or one use *Shi Quan Da Bu Tang* (Ten [Ingredients] Completely & Greatly Supplementing Decoction). If there is lower abdominal tension and pain and the menstruation is astringent and scanty, this can be combined with Radix Saussureae Seu Vladimiriae (*Mu Xiang*) and Rhizoma Corydalis Yanhusuo (*Yan Hu Suo*).

Kidney Vacuity

One should supplement and boost the liver and kidneys, nourish the blood and regulate the menstruation. The formula to use is *Dang Gui Di Huang Yin* (Dang Gui & Rehmannia Drink).

Blood Stasis

One should dispel stasis and quicken the blood. If stasis is dispelled, fresh blood will automatically be engendered. The formula to use is *Niu Xi Yin* (Achyranthes Drink). If there is simultaneous qi stagnation, use *Tao Hong Si Wu Tang* (Persica & Carthamus Four Materials Decoction) plus Pericarpium Citri Reticulatae (*Chen Pi*), Fructus Citri Sacrodactylis (*Fo Shou*), and Rhizoma Cyperi Rotundi (*Xiang Fu*).

49

Phlegm Dampness

One should dispel phlegm, transform dampness, and fortify the spleen. If phlegm dampness is eliminated, the spleen can obtain fortification and transportation. Thus the menstrual blood will automatically move correctly and come. The formula to use is *Xiong Gui Er Chen Tang* (Ligusticum & Dang Gui Two Aged [Ingredients] Decoction). Or one can use *Xiong Gui Er Chen Tang* plus Rhizoma Atractylodis (*Cang Zhu*) and Cortex Magnoliae Officinalis (*Hou Po*).

Explanation

This disease mostly manifests due to insufficiency of the source of engenderment and transformation. Therefore, its treatment should be mainly directed at the spleen and stomach. Xue Li-zhai says:

> Blood is the essence qi of water and grain. It harmonizes and regulates the five viscera. It sprinkles and moistens the six bowels. In men it is transformed into the essence. In women, above it becomes the breast milk. Below it becomes the menstrual water. Although the heart rules the blood and the liver stores the blood, the blood is also restrained and contained by the spleen. Therefore, supplementing the spleen and harmonizing the stomach results in automatically engendering the blood.

Thus one can see that scanty menstruation and spleen qi vacuity weakness not able to engender and transform the blood are closely connected. In clinical practice, one must necessarily use medicinals which can empower the spleen and stomach's transportation and transformation. However, when supplementing the blood, one should not use too many slimy, stagnating medicinals. It is also not permitted to recklessly use blood-breaking medicinals as such attack results in "vacating what is already vacuous."

Appended Formulas

1. *Si Wu Tang:* See Section One, same chapter.

2. *Shi Quan Da Bu Tang (*from *Tai Ping Hui Min He Ji Ju Fang [Tai Ping Imperial Grace Formulary]):* Radix Panacis Ginseng (*Ren Shen*), mix-fried Radix Astragali Membranacei (*Huang Qi*), scorched Rhizoma Atractylodis Macrocephalae (*Bai Zhu*), mix-fried Radix Glycyrrhizae (*Zhi Gan Cao*), Radix Angelicae Sinensis (*Dang Gui*), Radix Ligustici Wallichii (*Chuan Xiong*), prepared Radix Rehmanniae (*Shu Di*), Sclerotium Poriae Cocos (*Fu Ling*), Radix Albus Paeoniae Lactiflorae (*Bai Shao*), Cortex Cinnamomi (*Rou Gui*)

3. *Dang Gui Di Huang Yin* (from *Jing Yue Quan Shu (Jing-yue's Complete Writings]):* Radix Angelicae Sinensis (*Dang Gui*), prepared Radix Rehmanniae (*Shu Di*), Fructus Corni Officinalis (*Shan Zhu Yu*), Cortex Eucommiae Ulmoidis (*Du Zhong*), Radix Dioscoreae Oppositae (*Shan Yao*), Radix Achyranthis Bidentatae (*Niu Xi*), mix-fried Radix Glycyrrhizae (*Zhi Gan Cao*)

4. *Niu Xi Yin* (from *Ji Yin Gan Mu [Detailed Outline of Yin]):* Wine stir-fried Radix Achyranthis Bidentatae (*Niu Xi*), Cortex Cinnamomi (*Rou Gui*), Radix Rubrus Paeoniae Lactiflorae (*Chi Shao*), Semen Pruni Persicae (*Tao Ren*), Rhizoma Corydalis Yanhusuo (*Yan Hu Suo*), wine stir-fried Radix Angelicae Sinensis (*Dang Gui*), Radix Saussureae Seu Vladimiriae (*Mu Xiang*), Cortex Radicis Moutan (*Dan Pi*)

5. *Tao Hong Si Wu Tang* (from *Yi Zong Jin Jian [Golden Mirror of Ancestral Medicine]):* Prepared Radix Rehmanniae (*Shu Di*), Radix Angelicae Sinensis (*Dang Gui*), Radix Albus Paeoniae Lactiflorae (*Bai Shao*), Radix Ligustici Wallichii (*Chuan Xiong*), Semen Pruni Persicae (*Tao Ren*), Flos Carthami Tinctorii (*Hong Hua*)

6. *Xiong Gui Er Chen Tang:* See Section Two, same chapter.

Section Six

Painful Menstruation (*Tong Jing*)

If during, before, or after a woman's menstruation there is lower abdominal aching and pain or pain in the low back and sacrum, this is called painful menstruation or menstrual movement lower abdominal pain. If severe, the pain may be difficult to bear and commonly there is a somber white facial complexion, inversion chilling of the hands and feet, nausea and vomiting, headache and dizziness. If when the menstruation comes, one feels only a very faint lower abdominal distention, pain, and discomfort, this is considered normal and should not be treated as a disease.

Disease Causes, Disease Mechanisms

The disease mechanism of causing the onset of painful menstruation is mainly unsmooth or uneasy transportation and movement of the qi and blood. If there is no free flow, there is pain. If there is free flow, there is no pain. Non-smooth transportation and movement of the qi and blood may be due to the two causes of repletion and vacuity.

Repletion patterns are due to the emotions not being smooth. Liver qi thus becomes depressed and binds. The qi mechanism is inhibited. This results in the transportation and movement of the qi and blood being obstructed. This then produces qi stagnation and blood stasis and hence abdominal pain. Another cause is exposure to rain and immersion in water with invasion by cold dampness, eating and drinking chilled things, or sitting or lying on the damp earth. This can result in cold dampness invading the uterus. Cold evils cause the blood to congeal and stagnate. The menstrual blood is thus obstructed internally and hence the onset of menstrual pain.

Vacuity patterns are caused by qi and blood insufficiency. After the menstruation comes, the sea of blood is empty and vacuous and the *bao mai* loses its nourishment. It is also possible that the liver and kidneys may be constitutionally vacuous or that undisciplined bedroom affairs have caused detriment of the *chong* and *ren*. In that case, the essence is deficient and the blood is scanty and these are not able to enrich and nourish the *bao mai*. This then leads to the arising of menstrual movement pain.

In addition, liver depression/fire effulgence is categorized as heat and may also result in painful menstruation.

Disease Patterns

Qi Stagnation/Blood Stasis

One or two days before the period there occurs lower abdominal distention and pain which does not desire pressure. If qi stagnation is predominant, there is more distention and less pain. If blood stasis is predominant, there is more pain and less distention. The volume of the menses is astringent and scanty and its movement is not easy. The color of the menses is purple and dark or may contain clots. When these clots are expelled, the pain is reduced. There may also be chest, lateral costal, and breast distention and pain. The tongue is slightly dark or purple and dark and may have static spots. Its coating is thin. The pulse is deep and wiry or deep and choppy.

Cold Damp Congelation & Stagnation

Before or during menstruation there is chilly pain in the lower abdomen. If it obtains warmth, it is soothed. The volume of the menstruate is scanty and its movement is not smooth. Its color is dark red and it contains clots. The hands and feet are not warm, the tongue coating is white and slimy, and the pulse is deep and tight.

Qi & Blood Vacuity Weakness

At the time of or after menstruation there is an empty or insidious pain in the lower abdomen. There is a desire for both warmth and pressure. The volume is scanty, the color is pale, and the consistency is clear and watery. There is a somber white facial complexion, spiritual fatigue, lack of strength, a pale tongue with a thin, white coating, and a fine, weak pulse.

Liver/Kidney Deficiency Detriment

The amount of the menstruate is scanty and its color is pale. There is lower abdominal pain after the menstrual movement. There is also lower and upper back soreness, dizziness, tinnitus, a pale red tongue with a thin coating, and a deep, fine pulse.

Liver Depression/Fire Effulgence

The menses has not yet come, but there is commonly first aching and pain in the abdomen reaching both lateral costal regions. The volume of the menstruate is excessive and its color is purplish. There is also low back soreness, dizziness, flushed red face, irascibility, racing heart and palpitations during sleep, and red lips. The tongue is scarlet red with a scant coating, and the pulse is wiry and fine.

Treatment

Qi Stagnation/Blood Stasis

If there is mainly qi stagnation, one should course the liver and rectify the qi, assisted by quickening and nourishing the blood. The formula to use is *Jia Wei Wu Yao Tang* (Added Flavors Lindera Decoction) plus Radix Angelicae Sinensis (*Dang Gui*) and Radix Salviae Miltiorrhizae (*Dan Shen*) or *Ba Wu Tang*.

If there is mainly blood stasis, one should quicken the blood and move stasis, assisted by rectifying the qi and stopping pain. The formula to use is *Ge Xia Zhu Yu Tang* (Below the Diaphragm Dispel Stasis Decoction) or *Tao Hong Si Wu Tang* (Persica & Carthamus Four Materials Decoction) plus Rhizoma Corydalis Yanhusuo (*Yan Hu Suo*), Rhizoma Cyperi Rotundi (*Xiang Fu*), Herba Leonuri Heterophylli (*Yi Mu Cao*), and Radix Saussureae Seu Vladimiriae (*Mu Xiang*).

Cold Damp Congelation & Stagnation

One should warm the channels and scatter cold, dispel dampness and move stagnation. The formula to use is *Wu Zhu Yu Tang* (Evodia Decoction) or *Wen Jing Tang* (Warm the Menses Decoction) plus blast-fried Rhizoma Zingiberis (*Pao Jiang*), Radix Linderae Strychnifoliae (*Wu Yao*), and Semen Coicis Lachryma-jobi (*Yi Ren*).

Qi & Blood Vacuity Weakness

One should supplement the qi and nourish the blood. The formula to use is *Ba Zhen Yi Mu Tang* (Eight Pearls Leonurus Decoction) or *Sheng Yu Tang* (Sage-like Curing Decoction) plus Rhizoma Cyperi Rotundi (*Xiang Fu*) and Radix Glycyrrhizae (*Gan Cao*).

Liver/Kidney Deficiency Detriment

One should regulate and supplement the liver and kidneys. The formula to use is *Tiao Gan Tang* (Regulate the Liver Decoction).

Liver Depression/Fire Effulgence

One should level the liver and clear heat. The formula to use is *Xuan Yu Tong Jing Tang* (Diffuse Depression & Free the Flow of the Menses Decoction).

Explanation

1. The *Yi Zong Jin Jian (Golden Mirror of Ancestral Medicine)* says:

> If commonly there is abdominal pain with menstruation but the pain comes after the menstruation, this is due to qi and blood vacuity weakness. If the pain precedes the menses, this is qi and blood stasis and stagnation. If due to qi stagnating the blood, mostly there is distention and fullness. If due to blood stagnating the qi, mostly there is aching and pain. Thus treatment should be based on whether there is stasis or stagnation,

distention or pain, and whether this is due to vacuity or repletion, heat or cold.

Therefore, depending upon the time the aching and pain occur and the nature of the aching and pain, painful periods are discriminated according to cold, heat, vacuity, and repletion. Typically, aching and pain before or during the menstruation are replete, and pain after the menstruation is vacuous. Pain which refuses pressure is categorized as replete; pain which likes pressure is categorized as vacuity. If the obtainment of heat diminishes the pain, this is cold. If the obtainment of heat aggravates the pain, this is heat. If pain is more severe than distention and, when blood clots are expelled, the pain diminishes, this is stasis. If distention is more severe than pain, this is stagnation. Wrenching, chilly pain is categorized as cold. Piercing pain is categorized as heat. Insidious pain or tense pain is vacuity. These are the key points in the clinical discrimination of patterns in painful menstruation.

2. In the treatment of painful menstruation, nourishing the blood and rectifying the qi should be equally emphasized. The majority of cases with premenstrual pain are due to qi stagnation and blood stasis. Therefore, one should mainly rectify the qi, aided by nourishing the blood. However, most postmenstrual pain is caused by blood vacuity with qi stagnation. Therefore, nourishing the blood is the chief, assisted by rectifying the qi. Based on clinical experience, *Ai Fu Si Wu Tang* (Mugwort & Aconite Four Materials Decoction) plus Cortex Cinnamomi (*Rou Gui*) is quite effective in the treatment of blood vacuity and qi stagnation when accompanied by cold. However, prepared Radix Rehmanniae (*Shu Di*) should be prepared with Fructus Amomi (*Sha Ren*). If the tongue coating is white and slimy, delete prepared Radix Rehmanniae (*Shu Di*) and add transforming dampness medicinals. If there has been excessive reproduction or excessive loss of blood, add Fructus Evodiae Rutecarpae (*Wu Zhu Yu*) and Fructus Foeniculi Vulgaris (*Xiao Hui Xiang*) for better results. If there is painful menstruation and early menstruation due to qi stagnation and blood heat, use *Xiao Yao San* (Rambling Powder) plus Rhizoma Cyperi Rotundi (*Xiang Fu*), Rhizoma Corydalis Yanhusuo (*Yan Hu Suo*), Cortex Radicis Moutan (*Dan Pi*), and Radix Albus Paeoniae Lactiflorae (*Bai Shao*) for best results.

3. Radix Angelicae Sinensis (*Dang Gui*), Rhizoma Corydalis Yanhusuo (*Yan Hu Suo*), and Radix Albus Paeoniae Lactiflorae (*Bai Shao*) are three essential ingredients for all types of painful menstruation. Other ingredients can be added accordingly. For example, if there is pain on both sides of the lower abdomen, add Fructus Foeniculi Vulgaris (*Xiao Hui Xiang*) and Semen Citri Reticulatae (*Ju He*).

4. Another clinically encountered variation of painful menstruation is caused by the fact that the wrapper network vessels (*bao luo*) are empty and vacuous after menstruation, delivery, or miscarriage. Evil toxins (*i.e.*, wind heat or damp heat evils) may taking advantage of vacuity and invade, thus causing the appearance of painful periods. This is quite similar to pelvic inflammatory disease or endometritis in modern medicine. Symptoms seen in that case include lower abdominal distention and pain possibly extending to the lower back and thighs, fever, and excessive vaginal discharge before the menses which is either yellow or red and white and has a foul odor. The menstruate is excessive in volume and contains clots. The tongue coating is yellow and slimy, and the pulse is wiry and rapid. Correspondingly, one should clear heat and transform dampness, course the liver and dispel stasis. One can use *Xiao Yao San* (Rambling Powder) plus *Ju He Wan* (Orange Seed Pills) plus the addition of Caulis Sargentodoxae (*Hong Teng*), Herba Patriniae Heterophyllae (*Bai Jiang Cao*), Caulis Lonicera (*Ren Dong Teng*), and Fructus Gardeniae Jasminoidis (*Zhi Zi*). If blood stasis predominates, one can use *Xue Fu Zhu Yu Tang* (Blood Mansion Dispel Stasis Decoction) plus Semen Coicis Lachryma-jobi (*Yi Yi Ren*), Caulis Sargentodoxae (*Hong Teng*), Herba Patriniae Heterophyllae (*Bai Jiang Cao*), and Fructus Meliae Toosendan (*Chuan Lian Zi*).

5. As for patent medicines for painful menstruation, if there is qi stagnation and blood stasis with more distention than pain, one can use *Qi Zhi Xiang Fu Wan* (Seven Times Processed Cyperus Pills). If one has more pain than distention, one can administer *Yi Mu Gao* (Leonurus Paste). If there is cold dampness congealing and stagnating, one can administer *Yi Kun Jin Ku Jin Dan* (Boost *Kun* [*i.e.*, Earth], Save Bitterness Elixir). If there is qi and blood vacuity weakness, one can administer *Ba Zhen Yi Mu Wan* (Eight

Pearls Leonurus Pills) or *Ba Bao Kun Shun Dan* (Eight Treasures, Normalize *Kun* Elixir). If there is liver/kidney yin deficiency, one can administer *Huang Jing Dan* (Solomon's Seal Elixir). If there is liver depression/fire effulgence, one can administer *Dan Zhi Xiao Yao Wan* (Moutan & Gardenia Rambling Pills).

Appended Formulas

1. *Jia Wei Wu Yao Tang* (from *Zheng Zhi Zhun Sheng [Patterns & Treatments Norms & Criteria]*): Radix Linderae Strychnifoliae (*Wu Yao*), Fructus Amomi (*Sha Ren*), Radix Saussureae Seu Vladimiriae (*Mu Xiang*), Rhizoma Corydalis Yanhusuo (*Yan Hu Suo*), Rhizoma Praeparata Cyperi, mix-fried Radix Glycyrrhizae (*Zhi Gan Cao*), uncooked Rhizoma Zingiberis (*Sheng Jiang*)

2. *Ba Wu Tang* (Wang Hai-zang's formula): Radix Angelicae Sinensis (*Dang Gui*), Radix Ligustici Wallichii (*Chuan Xiong*), Radix Albus Paeoniae Lactiflorae (*Bai Shao*), Rhizoma Corydalis Yanhusuo (*Yan Hu Suo*), Fructus Meliae Toosendan (*Chuan Lian Zi*), Radix Saussureae Seu Vladimiriae (*Mu Xiang*), Semen Arecae Catechu (*Bing Lang*), prepared Radix Rehmanniae (*Shu Di*)

3. *Ge Xia Zhu Yu Tang* (from *Yi Lin Gai Cuo [Corrections of Mistakes in the Medical Forest]*): Radix Angelicae Sinensis (*Dang Gui*), Cortex Radicis Moutan (*Dan Pi*), Radix Ligustici Wallichii (*Chuan Xiong*), Semen Pruni Persicae (*Tao Ren*), Flos Carthami Tinctorii (*Hong Hua*), Fructus Citri Seu Ponciri (*Zhi Ke*), Rhizoma Corydalis Yanhusuo (*Yan Hu Suo*), Feces Trogopterori Seu Pteromi (*Wu Ling Zhi*), Cortex Radicis Moutan (*Dan Pi*), Rhizoma Cyperi Rotundi (*Xiang Fu*), Radix Linderae Strychnifoliae (*Wu Yao*), Radix Glycyrrhizae (*Gan Cao*)

4. *Tao Hong Si Wu Tang:* See Section Five, same chapter.

5. *Wen Jing Tang* (from *Fu Ren Da Quan Liang Fang [Great Complete {Collection of} Fine Formulas for Women]*): Radix Angelicae Sinensis (*Dang Gui*), Radix Ligustici Wallichii (*Chuan Xiong*), Radix Albus

Paeoniae Lactiflorae (*Bai Shao*), Rhizoma Curcumae Zedoariae (*E Zhu*), Radix Panacis Ginseng (*Ren Shen*), Radix Achyranthis Bidentatae (*Niu Xi*), Cortex Cinnamomi (*Rou Gui*), Cortex Radicis Moutan (*Dan Pi*), mix-fried Radix Glycyrrhizae (*Zhi Gan Cao*)

6. *Wu Zhu Yu Tang* (from *Zheng Zhi Zhun Sheng [Patterns & Treatments Norms & Criteria]*): Fructus Evodiae Rutecarpae (*Dan Wu Zhu*), Radix Angelicae Sinensis (*Dang Gui*), Radix Platycodi Grandiflori (*Jie Geng*), Herba Cum Radice Asari Seiboldi (*Xi Xin*), Radix Ledebouriellae Sesloidis (*Fang Feng*), dry Rhizoma Zingiberis (*Gan Jiang*), prepared Radix Rehmanniae (*Shu Di*), mix-fried Radix Glycyrrhizae (*Zhi Gan Cao*)

7. *Ba Zhen Yi Mu Tang* (from *Ji Sheng Fang [Formulas for the Aid of the Living]*): Herba Leonuri Heterophylli (*Yi Mu Cao*), Radix Panacis Ginseng (*Ren Shen*), Rhizoma Atractylodis Macrocephalae (*Bai Zhu*), Sclerotium Poriae Cocos (*Fu Ling*), Radix Glycyrrhizae (*Gan Cao*), Radix Angelicae Sinensis (*Dang Gui*), prepared Radix Rehmanniae (*Shu Di*), Radix Ligustici Wallichii (*Chuan Xiong*), Radix Albus Paeoniae Lactiflorae (*Bai Shao*)

8. *Sheng Yu Tang* (from *Lan Shi Mi Cang [Secrets from the Orchid Chamber]*): Radix Codonopsis Pilosulae (*Dang Shen*), Radix Astragali Membranacei (*Huang Qi*), Radix Angelicae Sinensis (*Dang Gui*), prepared Radix Rehmanniae (*Shu Di*), Radix Albus Paeoniae Lactiflorae (*Bai Shao*), Radix Ligustici Wallichii (*Chuan Xiong*)

9. *Tiao Gan Tang* (from *Fu Qing Zhu Nu Ke [Fu Qing-zhu's Gynecology]*): Radix Angelicae Sinensis (*Dang Gui*), stir-fried Radix Albus Paeoniae Lactiflorae (*Bai Shao*), stir-fried Radix Dioscoreae Oppositae (*Shan Yao*), stir-fried Gelatinum Corii Asini (*E Jiao*), Fructus Corni Officinalis (*Shan Zhu Yu*), saltwater stir-fried Radix Morindae Officinalis (*Ba Ji Tian*), Radix Glycyrrhizae (*Gan Cao*)

10. *Xuan Yu Tong Jing Tang* (from *Fu Qing Zhu Nu Ke [Fu Qing-zhu's Gynecology]*): Radix Angelicae Sinensis (*Dang Gui*), stir-fried Radix Albus Paeoniae Lactiflorae (*Bai Shao*), Cortex Radicis Moutan (*Dan Pi*),

59

scorched Fructus Gardeniae Jasminoidis (*Zhi Zi*), stir-fried Semen Sinapis Albae (*Bai Jie Zi*), Radix Bupleuri (*Chai Hu*), processed Rhizoma Cyperi Rotundi (*Xiang Fu*), Tuber Curcumae (*Yu Jin*), stir-fried Radix Scutellariae Baicalensis (*Huang Qin*), uncooked Radix Glycyrrhizae (*Gan Cao*)

Section Seven

Menstrual Movement Epistaxis (*Jing Xing Tu Nu*)

One or two days before the menstruation comes, on the day the menses is scheduled to come, or instead of the menses which do not come, one may experience the onset of epistaxis with blood discharging from the nose. This is called menstrual movement epistaxis. It is also called counterflow menstruation or moving about (*i.e.*, vicarious) menstruation.

Disease Causes, Disease Mechanisms

This disease's causes can be divided into two types:

1. Blood Heat Reckless Movement

This is mostly due to overeating acrid, hot, agitating substances or due to constitutional yin deficiency with fire effulgence. There is heat in the blood aspect and fire qi upbears above. The *Fu Ke Mi Jue Da Quan (Great Complete [Collection of] Secrets of Success in Gynecology)* says: "If a woman's menses moves about, this is due to blood heat and fire qi moving upward."

2. Liver Qi Counterflowing Upward

This is due to the liver's impetuous nature. Normal flow is appropriate, but counterflow is not appropriate. Normal flow leads to quiet. Counterflow leads to qi stirring. Since blood follows the qi, it moves upward. Qi counterflow leads to blood recklessly stirring and this produces moving about menstruation.

More often than not, the above two causes present simultaneously. It is obvious that the primary cause of this disorder is kidney water insufficiency. This leads easily to blood heat recklessly moving and liver qi counterflowing upward. As Zhang Shan-lei says:

> In moving about menstruation, there is upbearing but no downbearing. Perverse movement counterflows. This is mostly due to kidney vacuity below with yang thus rising upward.

However, moving about menstruation with oral or nasal bleeding is not actually menstrual blood moving about. Rather, it is blood heat and liver counterflow damaging the network vessels resulting in bleeding. Because the amount of menstruation decreases or because the menstruation may fail to appear when there is nasal bleeding, this is often interpreted as the menstrual water which fire and heat have simmered and boiled and which thus have become dry and scanty.

Disease Patterns

Blood Heat Reckless Movement

One or two days or just when the menstruation comes, there is sudden hemoptysis or epistaxis, while the volume of the menses is scanty. It is also possible for the menses to stop and not come. There is abdominal pain, dry mouth and throat, flushed red cheeks, heart vexation, no sleep, a red tongue with a scant coating, and a fine, rapid pulse.

Liver Qi Counterflowing Upward

Before or during the menstruation there is hemoptysis or epistaxis with heart vexation, easy anger, distention and pain of the two lateral costal regions, a bitter taste in the mouth, and dry throat. If the blood discharged

61

is excessive, then the face has a scant blood color. The tongue is red with a thin, yellow coating, and the pulse is wiry and rapid.

Treatment

Blood Heat Reckless Movement

One should clear heat, cool the blood, and enrich yin. The formula to use is *Qing Gan Yin Jing Tang* (Clear the Liver & Conduct the Menses Decoction). If replete heat is heavy and bleeding is excessive, the formula to use is *San Huang Si Wu Tang* (Three Yellows Four Materials Decoction) or *Xi Jiao Di Huang Tang* (Rhinoceros Horn & Rehmannia Decoction) with additions and subtractions.

Liver Qi Counterflowing Upward

One should level the liver and normalize the flow of the menses. The formula to use is *Shun Jing Tang* (Normalize the Flow of the Menses Decoction).

Explanation

1. Most patients with this disease are young women or unmarried women who are mostly discriminated as blood heat and repletion. Therefore, typically treatment is to clear heat and cool the blood, assisted by enriching yin and harmonizing and freeing the flow of the menstruation medicinals, and this achieves good results. However, overdosage of securing and astringent ingredients and those which are bitter and cold should be avoided or these will damage the spleen and stomach.

2. Those with this disease are prohibited to eat acrid, hot foods, such as peppers, fresh ginger, onions and garlic, and alcohol. They should also continuously try to avoid emotional disturbance.

Appended Formulas

1. *Qing Gan Yin Jing Tang* (from *Zhong Yi Fu Ke Xue [The Study of TCM Gynecology]):* Radix Angelicae Sinensis (*Dang Gui*), Radix Albus Paeoniae Lactiflorae (*Bai Shao*), uncooked Radix Rehmanniae (*Sheng Di*), Cortex Radicis Moutan (*Dan Pi*), Fructus Gardeniae Jasminoidis (*Zhi Zi*), Radix Scutellariae Baicalensis (*Huang Qin*), Fructus Meliae Toosendan (*Chuan Lian Zi*), Radix Rubiae Cordifoliae (*Qian Cao*), Rhizoma Imperatae Cylindricae (*Bai Mao Gen*), Radix Achyranthis Bidentatae (*Niu Xi*), Radix Glycyrrhizae (*Gan Cao*)

2. *San Huang Si Wu Tang* (from *Yi Zong Jin Jian (Golden Mirror of Ancestral Medicine]):* Radix Angelicae Sinensis (*Dang Gui*), uncooked Radix Rehmanniae (*Sheng Di*), Radix Albus Paeoniae Lactiflorae (*Bai Shao*), Radix Ligustici Wallichii (*Chuan Xiong*), Radix Scutellariae Baicalensis (*Huang Qin*), Rhizoma Coptidis Chinensis (*Huang Lian*)

3. *Xi Jiao Di Huang Tang* (from *Qian Jin Yao Fang [Essential Formulas {Worth a} Thousand {Pieces of} Gold]):* Cornu Rhinocerotis (*Xi Jiao*, substitute Cornu Bubali [*Shui Niu Jiao*]), uncooked Radix Rehmanniae (*Sheng Di*), Radix Rubrus Paeoniae Lactiflorae (*Chi Shao*), Cortex Radicis Moutan (*Dan Pi*)

4. *Shun Jing Tang* (from *Fu Qing Zhu Nu Ke [Fu Qing-zhu's Gynecology]):* Radix Angelicae Sinensis (*Dang Gui*), prepared Radix Rehmanniae (*Shu Di*), Radix Albus Paeoniae Lactiflorae (*Bai Shao*), Cortex Radicis Moutan (*Dan Pi*), Sclerotium Poriae Cocos (*Fu Ling*), Radix Glehniae Littoralis (*Sha Shen*), blackened Herba Seu Flos Schizonepetae Tenuifoliae (*Jie Sui*)

Section Eight

Menstrual Movement Breast Distention & Pain (*Jing Xing Ru Fang Zhang Tong*)

Breast distention and pain may occur before or during menstruation. If severe, the pain cannot bear even the slightest pressure. This is called menstrual movement breast distention and pain. If this disease is recurrent and left uncured, this may lead to the arising of infertility or mammary neoplasia.

Disease Causes, Disease Mechanisms

The breasts are traversed by the foot *yang ming* stomach channel and network vessels, while a network vessel of the foot *jue yin* liver channel homes to the nipple. Therefore, the onset of this disease is closely related to the two channels of the liver and stomach. Hence, liver depression and qi stagnation or liver/stomach depressive fire may lead to menstrual movement breast distention and pain. Liver depression/qi stagnation causes loss of normalcy in coursing and discharge. The channels and vessels are inhibited and this leads to the arising of breast distention and thence to pain. Liver/stomach depressive fire causes brewing and binding which transforms into heat and fire. Fire qi stirs internally which follows the channels and causes pain. The network vessels of the breasts are injured and burnt. Hence the nipple is itchy and there is breast distention and pain or burning heat aching and pain.

Disease Patterns

Liver Depression/ Qi Stagnation

There is premenstrual distention or pain or there may be nodulations. Pain radiates to the chest and lateral costal regions. There is also lower

64

abdominal distention and pain, emotional depression, possible painful menstruation or possible infertility. The tongue is slightly dark with a thin coating, and the pulse is wiry.

Liver/Stomach Depressive Fire

There is menstrual movement piercing pain in the breast and nipple itching, possible flowing yellow water, burning heat in the breasts, heart vexation, easy anger, a dry mouth, chest and lateral costal distention and oppression, dizziness, and tinnitus. There may also be infertility and abnormal vaginal discharge. The tongue is red with a dry, yellow coating, and the pulse is wiry and rapid.

Treatment

Liver Depression/Qi Stagnation

One should course the liver and rectify the qi, assisted by opening the network vessels. The formula to use is *Xiao Yao San* (Rambling Powder) plus Pericarpium Viridis Citri Reticulatae (*Qing Pi*), Pericarpium Citri Reticulatae (*Chen Pi*), Folium Citri Reticulatae (*Ju Ye*), Fructus Liquidambaris Taiwaniae (*Lu Lu Tong*), and Semen Citri Reticulatae (*Ju He*). If the pain is severe, add Resina Olibani (*Ru Xiang*), Resina Myrrhae (*Mo Yao*), and Rhizoma Corydalis Yanhusuo (*Yan Hu Suo*). If there are painful breast lumps, add Squama Manitis Pentadactylis (*Chuan Shan Jia*) and Semen Vaccariae Segetalis (*Wang Bu Liu Xing*). If the breast is obviously enlarged, add Caulis Aristolochiae (*Tian Xian Teng*).

Liver/Stomach Depressive Fire

One should clear heat and drain fire, aided by resolving depression. the formula to use is *Dan Zhi Xiao Yao San* (Moutan & Gardenia Rambling Powder) from which Sclerotium Poriae Cocos (*Fu Ling*) and Rhizoma Atractylodis Macrocephalae (*Bai Zhu*) have been omitted and to which

65

Spica Prunellae Vulgaris (*Xia Ku Cao*), Radix Scutellariae Baicalensis (*Huang Qin*), Radix Trichosanthis Kirlowii (*Tian Hua Fen*), Herba Cum Radice Taraxaci Mongolici (*Pu Gong Ying*), and uncooked Radix Rehmanniae (*Sheng Di*) have been added. If there is heart vexation and insomnia, add Cortex Albizziae Julibrissinis (*He Huan Pi*). If there is excessive vaginal discharge with a foul odor, add Cortex Phellodendri (*Huang Bai*), Rhizoma Smilacis Glabrae (*Tu Fu Ling*), and Cortex Ailanthi Altissimi (*Chun Gen Pi*). If there are hard lumps which do not disperse, add Thallus Algae (*Kun Bu*) and Herba Sargassii (*Hai Zao*).

Explanation

This disease is commonly seen in clinical practice and often seen in those with infertility. Nevertheless, treatment with Chinese medicinals can achieve good results with menstrual movement breast distention and pain and can also help cure infertility.

Appended Formulas

1. *Xiao Yao San:* See Section Two, same chapter.

2. *Dan Zhi Xiao Yao San:* See Section Two, Chapter Six.

Section Nine

Menstrual Block (*Jing Bi*)

If, in females above 18 years of age, menstruation has never come like a tide or has come regularly but then has stopped for more than 3 months, and if there are other associated signs and symptoms, this is called blocked menstruation or amenorrhea. Menstruation which has stopped during pregnancy, during lactation, or after menopause is a normal physiological manifestation and is not categorized as menstrual block. If prenatally a woman does not have a uterus, ovaries, vaginal tract, or does have an unperforated hymen, although all these pathological conditions may result in menstrual block, they cannot be treated with herbal medicinals. Therefore, they are beyond the scope of this present discussion.

Disease Causes, Disease Mechanism

This disease is mainly divided into the two types of blood stagnation menstrual block and blood withering menstrual block. There are also a few who may have phlegm obstruction menstrual block.

Blood stagnation menstrual block is divided into the two causes of qi depression causing stagnation and wind chill stasis and binding. Qi depression causing stagnation is mostly due to worry, (excessive) thinking, irritation, and anger or by fright, fear and grief. These lead to the qi mechanism not being smoothly flowing. Blood stagnates internally and does not move. Wind chill stasis and binding is due to habitual preference for or eating during the menses sour, chilly foods, melons and fruits. It may also be due to invasion by cold and chill externally during the menstruation. This leads to congelation and binding below and the production of stasis and eventually block and binding.

Blood withering menstrual block is due to insufficiency of the source of menstrual blood. This, in turn, may be due to heat drying or to spleen and kidney vacuity blood deficiency. In the case of heat drying, if it endures, it undoubtedly causes tidal fever. Fluids and blood are thus dispersed and consumed. Thus the blood becomes withered and does not move. In the case of spleen vacuity, due to damage and detriment of the spleen and stomach, food and drink are decreased and thus do not transform essence and engender blood. Therefore the blood vessels' flow becomes withered. If there is kidney vacuity blood deficiency, this is due to the aftermath of blood loss or excessive births and breast-feeding. It may also be due to excessive bedroom taxation or due to heart/lung detriment which leads to the blood and fluids becoming dry. This thus produces menstrual block or amenorrhea.

Phlegm obstruction menstrual block is due to spleen yang not transporting. Phlegm dampness obstructs internally. It is also possible that habitual preference for oily, slimy, thick-flavored foods transforms and engenders phlegm turbidity. This then obstructs and stagnates in the *chong* and *ren*. The *bao mai* thus becomes blocked and hindered and this results in menstrual block and non-movement. Clinically, this is mostly seen in obese women. As the *Nu Ke Qie Yao (Immediate Essentials of Gynecology)* says, "Fat women with menstrual block must necessarily have phlegm dampness and fatty tissue congesting and hindering."

Disease Patterns

Blood Stagnation Menstrual Block: This can be discriminated into two patterns as described below.

Qi Depression Causing Stagnation

There is emotional depression, dizziness, headache, chest and lateral costal distention and pain, devitalized appetite, low back soreness, and abnormal vaginal discharge. The menstruation becomes progressively more chaotic and eventually this becomes menstrual block. The tongue coating is white and slimy, and the pulse image is wiry and fine.

Wind Chill Stasis & Binding

There is menstrual block with abdominal pain and distention which does not desire pressure. There is also abnormal vaginal discharge, low back soreness, a somber, and dark or bluish white facial complexion. If there are cold evils, the body is also cold, there is aversion to cold, and there is headache and stiff neck. The tongue is dark red or has purple patches or spots. The pulse image is deep and choppy or deep, slow, and tight.

Blood Withering Menstrual Block: This may be divided into the following three disease cause patterns.

Heat Drying

There is Heart vexation, scorching agitation, afternoon tidal fever, a bitter taste in the mouth, dry throat, bodily emaciation, dry, bound stool, scant, and reddish urine. The menstruation progressively goes from being from early to being scanty to eventually becoming menstrual block. The tongue is scarlet and may have either a thin, dry, yellow coating or a flowery, peeled coating. The pulse is wiry, fine, and rapid.

Spleen Vacuity

The menses are pale in color and scanty in volume. Delayed menstruation eventually becomes menstrual block the facial complexion is somber yellow. There is essence spirit fatigue, clear chill of the four limbs, dizziness, lack of strength, heart palpitations, shortness of breath, reduced food intake, occasional abdominal distention, loose stools, a white, slimy tongue coating, and a vacuous fine, slow pulse.

Kidney Vacuity

There is tidal fever in the afternoon, vexatious heat in the bones and flesh of the hands and feet, dizziness, heart palpitations, low back soreness, upper back pain, possible cough and night sweats, shortness of breath and bodily emaciation, and a somber white facial complexion. The pulse is deep, vacuous, and rapid or fine, soft, and forceless. The tongue is pale or slightly scarlet.

Phlegm Obstruction Menstrual Block

The body is obese and the facial complexion is puffy and yellow. There is chest oppression, epigastric distention, diminished food intake, excessive phlegm, and abnormal vaginal discharge. The menses are pale in color and scanty, eventually turning into menstrual block. The tongue has a white, slimy coating, and the pulse image is wiry and slippery.

Treatment

Blood Stagnation Menstrual Block

Qi Depression Causing Stagnation

One should course the liver and open depression. The formula to use is *Xiao Yao San* (Rambling Powder) plus Semen Pruni Persicae (*Tao Ren*), Flos Carthami Tinctorii (*Hong Hua*), Cortex Radicis Moutan (*Dan Pi*), and Radix Achyranthis Bidentatae (*Niu Xi*). One can also use *Kai Yu Er Chen Tang* (Open Depression Two Aged [Ingredients] Decoction).

Wind Chill Stasis & Binding

One should dispel cold, warm the menses, and move the blood. the formula to use is *He Xue Tong Jing Tang* (Harmonize the Blood & Free the Flow of the Menses Decoction). If it is mostly an exterior pattern, one can use *Wu Zhu Yu Tang* (Evodia Decoction). If there concretions and conglomerations and mostly internal patterns, one can use *Hu Po San* (Succinum Powder), *Da Huang Zhe Chong Wan* (Rhubarb & Ophistho-platia Pills), or *Di Dang Tang* (Resistance Decoction).

Blood Withering Menstrual Block

Heat Drying

One should clear heat and nourish yin. The formula to use is *Di Huang Jian* (Rehmannia Decoction) or *Yi Guan Jian* (One Link Decoction).

Spleen Vacuity

One should supplement the spleen and boost the stomach, thus enriching the source of transformation. The formula to use is *Bu Zhong Yi Qi Tang Jia Jian* (Supplement the Center & Boost the Qi Decoction with Additions & Subtractions).

Kidney Vacuity

One should boost the kidneys and nourish the blood. If loss of blood has been excessive, use *Ren Shen Yang Rong Tang* (Ginseng Nourish the Constructive Decoction). If births or breast-feeding have been excessive, use *Shi Quan Da Bu Tang* (Ten [Ingredients] Completely & Greatly Supplementing Decoction). If there is excessive bedroom taxation, use *Liu Wei Di Huang Wan* (Six Flavors Rehmannia Pills). If there is heart/lung detriment, use *Yi Guan Jian* (One Link Decoction). And if there is blood vacuity with fire, use *Bai Zi Ren Wan* (Semen Biotae Pills).

Phlegm Obstruction Menstrual Block

One should transform phlegm and rectify dampness. The formula to use is *Cang Suo Dao Tan Wan* (Atractylodes & Cyperus Abduct Phlegm Pills) or *Hou Po Er Chen Tang* (Magnolia Two Aged [Ingredients] Decoction.

Explanation

1. It is important that, before one administers blood-breaking, attacking, and precipitating medicinals, one confirms or denies the suspicion of pregnancy in patients with menstrual block.

2. Likewise, menstrual block should be distinguished from bimonthly, quarterly and annual menstruation as well as occult menstruation. If the patient has always had a regular cycle, even at 2, 3, 4, or more months per cycle, this is not a symptom of disease and does not require treatment.

3. Because blood withering menstrual block is categorized as a vacuity pattern, one should mainly nourish the qi and blood. When the qi and blood are full and sufficient, the menstruation will automatically be free-flowing. It is not permissible to recklessly use blood-cracking medicinals. These may damage the righteous qi so severely as to cause greatly excessive uterine bleeding which will not stop. For spleen vacuity, it is appropriate to supplement the spleen and fortify the stomach. However, one should not

overuse enriching, slimy, supplementing medicinals. This will only cause obstruction which will check transportation and movement.

Appended Formulas

1. *Xiao Yao San:* See Section Two, same chapter.

2. *Kai Yu Er Chen Tang (*from *Wan Shi Fu Ke [Master Wan's Gynecology]):* Pericarpium Citri Reticulatae (*Chen Pi*), Sclerotium Poriae Cocos (*Fu Ling*), Rhizoma Atractylodis (*Cang Zhu*, Rhizoma Cyperi Rotundi (*Xiang Fu*), Radix Ligustici Wallichii (*Chuan Xiong*), Rhizoma Pinelliae Ternatae (*Ban Xia*), Pericarpium Citri Reticulatae (*Chen Pi*), Rhizoma Curcumae Zedoariae (*E Zhu*), Semen Arecae Catechu (*Bing Lang*), Radix Glycyrrhizae (*Gan Cao*), Radix Saussureae Seu Vladimiriae (*Mu Xiang*), uncooked Rhizoma Zingiberis (*Sheng Jiang*)

3. *He Xue Tong Jing Tang (*from *Wei Sheng Bao Jian [Precious Mirror of Defending Life]):* Radix Angelicae Sinensis (*Dang Gui*), prepared Radix Rehmanniae (*Shu Di*), Rhizoma Sparganii (*San Leng*), Rhizoma Curcumae Zedoariae (*E Zhu*), Radix Saussureae Seu Vladimiriae (*Mu Xiang*), Cortex Cinnamomi (*Rou Gui*), Flos Carthami Tinctorii (*Hong Hua*), Lignum Sappan (*Su Mu*), Sanguis Draconis (*Xue Jie*)

4. *Wu Zhu Yu Tang (*from *Yi Zong Jin Jian [Golden Mirror of Ancestral Medicine]):* Fructus Evodiae Rutecarpae (*Wu Zhu Yu*), Radix Angelicae Sinensis (*Dang Gui*), ginger(-processed) Rhizoma Pinelliae Ternatae (*Ban Xia*), Radix Ledebouriellae Sesloidis (*Fang Feng*), Radix Ligustici Wallichii (*Chuan Xiong*), Sclerotium Poriae Cocos (*Fu Ling*), Cortex Cinnamomi (*Rou Gui*), Cortex Radicis Moutan (*Dan Pi*), Tuber Ophiopogonis Japonicae (*Mai Dong*), Herba Cum Radice Asari Seiboldi (*Xi Xin*), dry Rhizoma Zingiberis (*Gan Jiang*), Radix Saussureae Seu Vladimiriae (*Mu Xiang*), mix-fried Radix Glycyrrhizae (*Zhi Gan Cao*)

5. *Hu Po San (*from *Lei Zheng Pu Ji Ben Shi Fang [Formulas of Universal Benefit from My Practice Arranged According to Patterns]):* Rhizoma

Sparganii (*San Leng*), Rhizoma Curcumae Zedoariae (*E Zhu*), Succinum (*Hu Po*), Radix Albus Paeoniae Lactiflorae (*Bai Shao*), Herba Artemisiae Anomalae (*Liu Ji Nu*), Cortex Radicis Moutan (*Dan Pi*), Cortex Cinnamomi (*Rou Gui*), Radix Linderae Strychnifoliae (*Wu Yao*), Rhizoma Corydalis Yanhusuo (*Yan Hu Suo*)

6. *Da Huang Zhe Chong Wan* (from *Jin Gui Yao Lue [Essentials from the Golden Cabinet]*): Radix Et Rhizoma Rhei (*Da Huang*), Radix Scutellariae Baicalensis (*Huang Qin*), Radix Glycyrrhizae (*Gan Cao*), Semen Pruni Persicae (*Tao Ren*), Semen Pruni Armeniacae (*Xing Ren*), Radix Albus Paeoniae Lactiflorae (*Bai Shao*), dry Radix Rehmanniae (*Di Huang*), Resina Rhi Vernicifulae (*Gan Qi*), Tabanus (*Meng Chong*), Hirudo (*Shui Zhi*), Holotrichia Diomphalia (*Qi Cao*), Eupolyphaga Seu Ophisthoplatia (*Zhe Chong*)

7. *Di Dang Tang* (from *Shang Han Lun [Treatise on Damage Due to Cold]*): Tabanus (*Meng Chong*), Hirudo (*Shui Zhi*), Radix Et Rhizoma Rhei (*Da Huang*), Semen Pruni Persicae (*Tao Ren*), pig's fat (*Zhu Zhi*)

8. *Di Huang Jian* (from *Quan Sheng Zhi Mi Fang [Whole Life Pointing Out Confusion Formulas]*): Pills made of 250g of juice of fresh uncooked Radix Rehmanniae (*Sheng Di*) boiled until it is reduced to about 120g. To this, add powered Radix Et Rhizoma Rhei (*Da Huang*). Take 9g with boiled water each time, 2 times per day.

9. *Yi Guan Jian*: See Section Two, same chapter.

10. *Ji Jian Bu Zhong Yi Qi Tang*: Radix Panacis Ginseng (*Ren Shen*), Rhizoma Atractylodis Macrocephalae (*Bai Zhu*), Radix Angelicae Sinensis (*Dang Gui*), Radix Astragali Membranacei (*Huang Qi*), Radix Albus Paeoniae Lactiflorae (*Bai Shao*), Radix Ligustici Wallichii (*Chuan Xiong*), Radix Bupleuri (*Chai Hu*), Pericarpium Citri Reticulatae (*Chen Pi*), Massa Medica Fermentata (*Shen Qu*), Fructus Germinatus Hordei Vulgaris (*Mai Ya*), dry Rhizoma Zingiberis (*Gan Jiang*), Fructus Zizyphi Jujubae (*Da Zao*)

11. *Ren Shen Yang Rong Tang (*from *Tai Ping Hui Min He Ji Ju Fang [Tai Ping Imperial Grace Formulary]):* See Section Two, same chapter.

12. *Shi Quan Da Bu Tang:* See Section Five, same chapter.

13. *Liu Wei Di Huang Wan* (Qian Yi's formula): Prepared Radix Rehmanniae (*Shu Di*), Fructus Corni Officinalis (*Shan Zhu Yu*), Radix Dioscoreae Oppositae (*Shan Yao*), Rhizoma Alismatis (*Ze Xie*), Cortex Radicis Moutan (*Dan Pi*), Sclerotium Poriae Cocos (*Fu Ling*)

14. *Bai Zi Ren Wan (*from *Fu Ren Da Quan Liang Fang [Great Complete {Collection of} Fine Formulas for Women)*: Semen Biotae Orientalis (*Bai Zi Ren*), Radix Achyranthis Bidentatae (*Niu Xi*), Herba Lycopi Lucidi (*Ze Lan*), Radix Dipsaci (*Chuan Xu Duan*), prepared Radix Rehmanniae (*Shu Di*), Herba Selaginellae Tamariscinae (*Juan Bo*)

15. *Cang Suo Dao Tan Wan (*from *Ye Tian Shi Nu Ke [Ye Tian-shi Gynecology])*: Rhizoma Atractylodis (*Cang Zhu*), infant's urine processed Rhizoma Cyperi Rotundi (*Xiang Fu*), Pericarpium Citri Reticulatae (*Chen Pi*), Sclerotium Poriae Cocos (*Fu Ling*), Fructus Citri Seu Ponciri (*Zhi Ke*), processed Rhizoma Pinelliae Ternatae (*Ban Xia*), Rhizoma Arisaematis (*Nan Xing*), mix-fried Radix Glycyrrhizae (*Zhi Gan Cao*), uncooked Rhizoma Zingiberis (*Sheng Jiang*)

16. *Hou Po Er Chen Tang* (Dan-xi's formula): Cortex Magnoliae Officinalis (*Hou Po*, Pericarpium Citri Reticulatae (*Chen Pi*), ginger(-processed) Rhizoma Pinelliae Ternatae (*Ban Xia*), Sclerotium Poriae Cocos (*Fu Ling*)

Section Ten

Uterine Bleeding (*Beng Lou*)

Uterine bleeding refers to irregular bleeding from the vaginal tract in women. Typically, if this is characterized by sudden onset and profuse quantity, it is called *beng* or flooding or flooding and strike (*beng zhong*). If it is marked by insidious onset and moderate blood loss, it is called *lou* or leakage or *lou xia*, leaking precipitation. Flooding is an acute condition, while leakage is a chronic one. Although flooding and leakage are divided into acute and chronic conditions, they nevertheless have the same disease mechanisms. In the course of development of this disease, these two often transform into each other. For instance, if there is enduring flooding which does not stop, qi and blood are consumed and become debilitated. This may then produce leakage. If enduring leakage does not stop, it may also develop into flooding. Thus clinically, flooding and leakage are usually seen in combination.

Disease Causes, Disease Mechanisms

The cause of this disease is mainly detriment and damage of the *chong* and *ren* which are not able to secure and contain the menstrual blood. As for the causes leading to such detriment and damage to the *chong* and *ren*, these are due to blood heat, damp heat, blood stasis, qi vacuity, and kidney vacuity as described below.

Blood Heat

Habitual or constitutional yang exuberance, over-eating acrid, peppery foods which assist yang, or excessive emotional excitement may cause liver fire accumulating internally. Hence blood heat moves recklessly.

Damp Heat

Enduring stagnation of damp heat and menstruation which is not cured for a long time forces the blood to move recklessly.

Blood Stasis

During menstruation or postpartum, if one has sexual affairs before the bleeding has ceased, this may cause detriment and damage to the *chong* and *ren*. Or during menstruation, external evils may invade and affect the *bao mai.* This results in blood stasis not being dispelled and fresh blood is not able to return to the channels. This then leads to the arising of flooding and leaking.

Qi Vacuity

Worry and anxiety beyond limit or overtaxation and fatigue may damage the spleen. This results in the spleen not being able to restrain the blood. The central qi is vacuous and debilitated and the sea of blood is not secured. The menstrual blood thus floods and leaks and precipitates downward.

Kidney Vacuity

Kidney qi insufficiency, early marriage, too many births, or bedroom taxation may damage the kidneys. The *chong* and *ren* do not secure and hence flooding and leakage are produced.

Disease Patterns

Blood Heat

There is sudden profuse uterine bleeding or menstrual leakage which does not stop for many days. Its color is deep red. The face is red and there is a dry mouth, vexation and agitation, scanty sleep, a red tongue with a yellow or scanty coating, and a slippery, rapid or fine and rapid pulse.

Damp Heat

Depending on whether excessive dampness or heat predominates, the symptoms are divided. If dampness is heavy, the precipitated blood is mixed with sticky fluids and soy-sauce-like water. The facial complexion is yellow or there may be superficial edema. There is heaviness of the head, dizziness and vertigo, essence spirit fatigue, chest oppression, epigastric glomus, and a pasty, slimy feeling inside the mouth. The tongue has a thin, white, slimy coating, and the pulse image is soggy and slippery.

If heat is heavy, the amount of the precipitated blood is excessive and its color is purplish. There is a foul odor and the consistency is thick and sticky. The facial complexion is red and there is possible fever, spontaneous perspiration, a bitter taste in the mouth, dry mouth, short, reddish urination, and constipation or loose stools which are not smoothly flowing. The tongue is red with a slimy, yellow coating, and the pulse is slippery and rapid.

Blood Stasis

The bleeding dribbles and drips without ceasing or suddenly precipitates in great amounts. Its color is purple and it contains clots. There is lower abdominal aching and pain which refuses pressure. After the blood clots are expelled, the pain is diminished. The tongue is purple and dark or the tips and edges have static spots. The pulse is deep and choppy.

Qi Vacuity

The precipitated blood is excessive in amount or dribbles and drips without cessation. Its color is pale red and its consistency is watery and thin. The facial complexion is somber white or there is vacuity edema. There is shortness of breath, disinclination to speak, essence spirit fatigue, scanty appetite, epigastric distention, and loose stools. The tongue is fat with a thin, white coating, and the pulse is fine and weak.

Kidney Vacuity

If kidney yin vacuity is predominant, the bleeding is scant or dribbles and drips without cessation. Its color is fresh red. This is accompanied by dizziness, tinnitus, vexatious heat in the five hearts, loss of sleep, low back soreness, a red tongue with a thin or absent coating, and a fine, rapid, forceless pulse.

If kidney yang vacuity predominates, the bleeding is excessive in amount or dribbles and drips without cessation. Its color is pale red. The essence spirit is devitalized, and there is head and eye vacuity vertigo, chilly limbs, fear of cold, low back and knee soreness and weakness, a dark, dull facial complexion, loose stools, long, clear urination, a pale tongue with a thin, white coating, and a deep, fine pulse.

Treatment

This disease's treatment methods correspond to the principles, "If acute, treat the branch; if chronic, treat the root." In the case of sudden, profuse uterine bleeding, one should first stop bleeding in order to prevent fainting due to excessive bleeding causing vacuity desertion. If bleeding is slight and relaxed, careful discrimination of patterns is necessary in order to find the root cause. After the bleeding is stopped, one should supplement the qi and blood in order to properly and completely deal with the root. Based on his personal clinical experience, Ye Tian-shi summarized this approach in the following three treatment principles: 1) stop bleeding, 2) seek the root, 3) secure the root. However, one cannot abandon proper differentiation and should apply these principles flexibly.

Blood Heat

One should clear heat and cool the blood, nourish the blood and stop bleeding. The formula to use is *Qing Re Gu Jing Tang* (Clear Heat & Secure the Menses Decoction) plus Radix Glehniae Littoralis (*Sha Shen*) and Tuber Ophiopogonis Japonicae (*Mai Dong*).

Damp Heat

If excessive heat is predominant, one should mainly clear heat assisted by dispelling dampness. The formula to use is *Jia Wei Dan Zhi Xiao Yao San* (Added Flavors Moutan & Gardenia Rambling Powder). If excessive dampness predominates, one should mainly dispel dampness assisted by clearing heat. The formula to use is *Sheng Yang Chu Shi Tang* (Upbear

Yang & Eliminate Dampness Decoction) plus Radix Scutellariae Baicalensis (*Huang Qin*) and carbonized Radix Sanguisorbae (*Di Yu*).

Blood Stasis

One should dispel stasis in order to stop bleeding. The formula to use is *Si Wu Tang* (Four Materials Decoction) and *Shi Xiao San* (Sudden Smile Powder) plus powdered Radix Pseudoginseng (*San Qi*), carbonized Radix Rubiae Cordifoliae (*Qian Cao*), and Gelatinum Corii Asini (*E Jiao*).

Qi Vacuity

One should supplement the spleen, boost the qi, and gather the blood in order to stop bleeding. The formula to use is either *Gui Pi Tang* (Restore the Spleen Decoction) or *Gu Ben Zhi Beng Tang* (Secure the Root & Stop Flooding Decoction) minus Radix Angelicae Sinensis (*Dang Gui*) but plus processed Radix Polygoni Multiflori (*Shou Wu*) and Os Sepiae Seu Sepiellae (*Hai Piao Xiao*).

Kidney Vacuity

If kidney yin vacuity predominates, one should enrich kidney yin. The formula to use is *Zuo Gui Wan* (Restore the Left [Kidney] Pills) minus Radix Achyranthis Bidentatae (*Niu Xi*) and Gelatinum Cornu Cervi (*Lu Jiao Jiao*), but adding Fructus Ligustri Lucidi (*Nu Zhen Zi*), Herba Ecliptae Prostratae (*Han Lian Cao*), and carbonized Cacumen Biotae Orientalis (*Ce Bai Ye*). Or one should foster yin and clear heat. In that case, the formula to use first is *Qing Re Gu Jing Tang* (Clear Heat & Secure the Menses Decoction). Afterwards use *Liu Wei Di Huang Wan* (Six Flavors Rehmannia Pills).

If kidney yang vacuity predominates, the formula to use is *You Gui Wan* (Restore the Right [Kidney] Pills) minus Cortex Cinnamomi (*Rou Gui*) and plus Radix Astragali Membranacei (*Huang Qi*), Radix Dipsaci (*Xu Duan*), Radix Polygoni Multiflori (*He Shou Wu*), blast-fried Rhizoma Zingiberis (*Pao Jiang*), and carbonized Radix Angelicae Sinensis (*Dang Gui*).

79

Explanation

1. If profuse uterine bleeding suddenly precipitates, patient must necessarily be alarmed and worried. Therefore, they should be treated according to the principles of "boosting the qi in blood desertion." For this, one can use *Du Sheng Tang* (Solitary Ginseng Decoction), *i.e.* 15-30g of Radix Panacis Ginseng (*Zhen Shen*). Quite often, as many as 3 packets of medicinals are prescribed per day, since 1 packet per day is useless in such serious cases. If there is serious yang vacuity blood desertion, the pulse should normally be fine and small. If it is surging and large, this is abnormal. In addition, attention should be paid to the condition of the stomach qi. If the stomach qi remains unharmed, even though the condition appears grave, it can obtain treatment. In other words, when using medicinals, one must take into account the spleen and stomach. Whether one is treating *beng* or *lou*, one should take this principle into account. Therefore, even though the uterine bleeding is due to heat, one should not use too many bitter, cold, stop bleeding medicinals or this will cause detriment and damage to the spleen and stomach. Thus the source of gathering the blood will not be able to reach and function and this makes treatment even more difficult.

2. In treating uterine bleeding, use of acrid, warm, stirring the blood medicinals, such as Radix Angelicae Sinensis (*Dang Gui*), should be handled with care. Radix Angelicae Sinensis is able to lead the blood and return it the channels. However, it is categorized as a yang within the blood medicinal which not only supplements but also quickens the blood. Therefore, it is best avoided in serious cases of *beng lou*. Even though it is an essential ingredient in a prescription, it is often replaced by other ingredients, such as carbonized Radix Angelicae Sinensis (*Gui Shen*), and *Du Sheng Tang* (Solitary Ginseng Decoction) is often substituted for *Dang Gui Bu Xue Tang* (Dang Gui Supplement the Blood Decoction). This is based on the idea of supplementing the qi in cases of blood desertion and preventing unfavorable actions aroused by Radix Angelicae Sinensis.

3. A number of ingredients for *beng lou* are used after being carbonized, since this process reinforces their hemostatic effect. The empirical

prescription *Shi Hui Wan* (Ten Ashes Pills) was created specifically based on this principle. If there is qi desertion, upbearing the qi medicinals should be stir-fried and carbonized, such as carbonized Rhizoma Cimicifugae (*Sheng Ma*) and Herba Seu Flos Schizonepetae Tenuifoliae (*Jing Jie*). For blood heat, cooling the blood medicinals can be stir-fried and carbonized, such as Cacumen Biotae Orientalis (*Ce Bai Ye*), Radix Sanguisorbae (*Di Yu*), and Radix Scutellariae Baicalensis (*Huang Qin*). For blood stasis, one can use, for instance, carbonized Pollen Typhae (*Pu Huang*). For qi stagnation, one can use vinegar stir-fried, carbonized Rhizoma Cyperi Rotundi (*Xiang Fu*). For blood cold, one can use, for instance, dry Rhizoma Zingiberis (*Gan Jiang*), stir-fried and carbonized. For blood desertion, one should astringe, Therefore, use Pulvis Fumi Carbonisatus (*Bai Cao Shuang*) and carbonized Petiolus Trachycarpi (*Zong Lu Tan*). However, carbonized medicinals may also have the side effect of the extravasated blood not being able to be precipitated smoothly. Therefore, carbonized medicinals should be administered with care, especially in those with *beng lou* and lower abdominal pain associated with qi stagnation and blood stasis.

4. Ye Tian-shi, a famous Qing Dynasty practitioner, treated *beng lou* in three broad steps: At the beginning of uterine bleeding, it is appropriate to stop bleeding in order to block the flow. As the uterine bleeding is stopping, it is appropriate to clear heat so as to settle the source. After uterine bleeding has stopped and the interior heat has been eliminated, it is appropriate to supplement the qi and blood in order to completely deal with the root. Blockage of hemorrhage means to stop bleeding. This is vitally important in treating sudden metrorrhagia. In such cases, delayed treatment or mismanagement may cause desertion and endanger the person's life. Settling or clearing the source means to treat the root. This is an important link in treating uterine bleeding. If due to this the bleeding has diminished or just dribbles and drips, then one must treat the root. Treatment of the root should correspond to the discrimination of patterns. It is not alright to misuse stop bleeding and heat-clearing formulas. This would be tantamount to vacating vacuity and causing repletion to be even more replete. Completely and properly treating the root means to secure the root. This is done by the methods of regulating and rectifying. Mostly this means

81

regulating and harmonizing the spleen and stomach since the spleen and stomach are the source of qi and blood engenderment and transformation. If, after uterine bleeding, one uses large formulas for enriching and supplementing, these may obstruct and check the qi mechanism, stagnate and slime the spleen and stomach. This will affect digestion adversely. Therefore, securing the root corresponds mainly to regulating and rectifying the spleen and stomach. When the middle burner is fortified and transporting, the source of engenderment and transformation recuperates. Only then can the effects of supplementation and boosting fully manifest.

5. At the time of profuse uterine bleeding, the patient should be instructed to absolutely stay in bed and to remain quiet. It is wise to lower the head and elevate the lower half of the body. In case of fainting, one can use the "carbonized vinegar black nose method." Burn a piece of charcoal or heat a steel weight until red hot and drop either of these in a container of vinegar. The steam produced by this heat will revive the patient and help restrain the bleeding. An alternative is to needle the point *Yin Tang* (M-HN-3).

6. Commonly, if older women have profuse uterine bleeding or if the menses resume like a flood after menopause, there may be a uterine tumor. It is essential that one check for this.

Appended Formulas

1. *Qing Re Gu Jing Tang (*from *Zhong Guo Fu Ke Bing Xue [A Study of Gynecological Diseases in China]):* Calcined Os Draconis (*Long Gu*), un-cooked Radix Rehmanniae (*Sheng Di*), stir-fried Radix Albus Paeoniae Lactiflorae (*Bai Shao*), Plastrum Testudinis (*Gui Ban*), calcined Concha Ostreae (*Mu Li*), stir-fried Fructus Gardeniae Jasminoidis (*Zhi Zi*), carbonized Radix Scutellariae Baicalensis (*Huang Qin*), stir-fried Gelatinum Corii Asini (*E Jiao*), carbonized Petiolus Trachycarpi (*Zong Pi*), carbonized Radix Sanguisorbae (*Di Yu*), Crinis Carbonisatus (*Xue Yu Tan*), Radix Panacis Quinquefolii (*Xi Yang Shen*)

2. *Jia Wei Dan Zhi Xiao Yao San* (from *Fu Qing Zhu Nu Ke [Fu Qing-zhu's Gynecology]*): Cortex Radicis Moutan (*Dan Pi*), blackened Fructus Gardeniae Jasminoidis (*Shan Zhi*), Radix Bupleuri (*Chai Hu*), Herba Menthae Haplocalysis (*Bo He*), Rhizoma Coptidis Chinensis (*Huang Lian*), Radix Scutellariae Baicalensis (*Huang Qin*), Rhizoma Atractylodis Macrocephalae (*Bai Zhu*), Radix Albus Paeoniae Lactiflorae (*Bai Shao*), Semen Biotae Orientalis (*Bai Zi Ren*), Radix Angelicae Sinensis (*Dang Gui*), Gelatinum Corii Asini (*E Jiao*), carbonized Radix Sanguisorbae (*Di Yu*), rice vinegar (*Mi Cu*), a small amount

3. *Sheng Yang Chu Shi Tang* (from *Pi Wei Lun [Treatise on the Spleen & Stomach]*): Rhizoma Cimicifugae (*Sheng Ma*), Radix Et Rhizoma Notopterygii (*Qiang Huo*), Radix Ledebouriellae Sesloidis (*Fang Feng*), Rhizoma Atractylodis (*Cang Zhu*), mix-fried Radix Glycyrrhizae (*Zhi Gan Cao*), Sclerotium Polypori Umbellati (*Zhu Ling*), Rhizoma Alismatis (*Ze Xie*), Fructus Alpiniae Oxyphyllae (*Yi Zhi Ren*), Rhizoma Pinelliae Ternatae (*Ban Xia*), Massa Medica Fermentata (*Shen Qu*), Fructus Germinatus Hordei Vulgaris (*Mai Ya*), Pericarpium Citri Reticulatae (*Chen Pi*)

4. *Shi Xiao San* (from *Tai Ping Hui Min He Ji Ju Fang [Tai Ping Imperial Grace Formulary]*): Pollen Typhae (*Pu Huang*), Feces Trogopterori Seu Pteromi (*Wu Ling Zhi*)

5. *Gui Pi Tang:* See Section One, same chapter.

6. *Gu Ben Zhi Beng Tang* (from *Fu Qing Zhu Nu Ke (Fu Qing-zhu's Gynecology)*: Radix Astragali Membranacei (*Huang Qi*), prepared Radix Rehmanniae (*Shu Di*), Rhizoma Atractylodis Macrocephalae (*Bai Zhu*), uncooked Rhizoma Zingiberis (*Sheng Jiang*), Radix Codonopsis Pilosulae (*Dang Shen*), Radix Angelicae Sinensis (*Dang Gui*)

7. *Zuo Gui Wan* (from *Jing Yue Quan Shu [Jing-yue's Complete Writings]*): Prepared Radix Rehmanniae (*Shu Di*), Fructus Corni Officinalis (*Shan Zhu Yu*), Fructus Lycii Chinensis (*Gou Qi Zi*), Gelatinum Cornu Cervi (*Lu Jiao Jiao*), Semen Cuscutae (*Tu Si Zi*), Radix Dioscoreae Oppositae (*Shan Yao*),

Gelatinum Plastri Testudinis (*Gui Ban Jiao*), Radix Achyranthis Bidentatae (*Huai Niu Xi*)

8. *Liu Wei Di Huang Wan:* See Section Nine, same chapter.

9. *You Gui Wan (*from *Jing Yue Quan Shu [Jing-yue's Complete Writings]):* Prepared Radix Rehmanniae (*Shu Di*), Radix Dioscoreae Oppositae (*Shan Yao*), Fructus Corni Officinalis (*Shan Zhu Yu*), Fructus Lycii Chinensis (*Gou Qi Zi*), Cortex Eucommiae Ulmoidis (*Du Zhong*), Semen Cuscutae (*Tu Si Zi*), Gelatinum Cornu Cervi (*Lu Jiao Jiao*), Radix Lateralis Praeparatus Aconiti Carmichaeli (*Fu Zi*), Radix Angelicae Sinensis (*Dang Gui*), Cortex Cinnamomi (*Rou Gui*)

Section Eleven

Menopausal Syndrome (*Jue Jing Qian Hou Zhu Zheng*)

At approximately fifty years of age in women, "The *ren mai* becomes vacuous, the *tai chong mai* become debilitated and scanty, and the *tian gui* is exhausted." Thus menstruation ceases at about this time. Although the menstruation around this time may be early, late, and erratic and its amount may be excessive or scanty, if there are no whole body symptoms, this is categorized as a normal physiological process. However, either before or after menopause, some women do experience a constellation of signs and symptoms. This is referred to as menopausal syndrome and climacteric syndrome. The clinical manifestations of this syndrome mostly include vexation, agitation, and easy anger, essence spirit fatigue, dizziness, heart palpitations, loss of sleep, a dry mouth and parched throat, no flavor for food, vexatious heat in the five hearts, tinnitus, poor memory, high blood pressure, low back soreness and upper back pain, skin itching, and, if severe, loss of normalcy of essence spirit (*i.e.*, mental/emotional disturbances). The severity and duration of these symptoms may vary greatly from case to case. If severe, they may last from 3-5 years.

Disease Causes, Disease Mechanisms

As the *Nei Jing (Inner Classic)* says:

> In women, at 7 years the kidney qi is exuberant...At 7x7, the *ren mai* is vacuous, the *tai chong mai* has become debilitated and scanty, and the *tian gui* is exhausted. Thus the pathways are not open, the body is spoilt, and there are no more children.

Therefore, around the age of 49 in women, the kidney qi declines, the *chong* and *ren* become deficient and suffer detriment. The *tian gui* ceases, the essence spirit is insufficient, and yin and yang lose their balance. Hence, there appear various signs of loss of regulation of yin and yang. Kidney yin vacuity may not subdue yang which loses its treasuring, or kidney yang may be vacuous and debilitated and the channels and vessels may lose their warmth and nourishment. This may eventually lead to the loss of normalcy of the functions of the other viscera and bowels. Based on the above analysis, kidney vacuity is the root cause of this disease. In addition, there may also be heart/spleen dual vacuity resulting in loss of regulation of the qi and blood and thus the *chong* and *ren*, giving rise to the appearance of menopausal syndrome.

Disease Patterns

Liver/Kidney Yin Vacuity

Water deficiency leads to fire effulgence. Therefore there is booming heat (*i.e.*, hot flashes) with sweating, heart vexation, easy anger, vexatious heat in the five hearts, dizziness, headache, loss of sleep, tinnitus, low back and knee soreness and weakness, dry mouth, constipation, a red tongue with scanty coating, and a fine, rapid pulse.

Kidney Yang Vacuity & Debility

The facial complexion is somber white. There is fear of cold, chilled limbs, spiritual fatigue, low back soreness, clear, long urination or scanty

85

urination with superficial edema. The tongue is pale with a thin, white coating. The pulse is deep, fine, and forceless.

Kidney Yin & Yang Dual Vacuity

There is dizziness, vertigo, tinnitus, low back soreness, lack of strength, lack of warmth in the four limbs, sometimes possible dread of chill, sometimes booming heat. The tongue is pale and the pulse is deep, fine, and wiry.

Heart/Spleen Dual Vacuity

There are heart palpitations, shortness of breath, poor memory, loss of sleep, a sallow yellow facial complexion, fatigue, lack of strength, scanty appetite, slight epigastric and abdominal distention, superficial edema of the face, eyes, and four limbs, a pale tongue with a thin coating, and a fine, soggy pulse.

Treatment

Liver/Kidney Yin Vacuity

On should enrich yin and downbear fire, boost the kidneys and subdue yang. The formula to use is *Zhi Bai Di Huang Tang* (Anemarrhena & Phellodendron Rehmannia Pills) plus Os Draconis (*Long Gu*) and Concha Ostreae (*Mu Li*). Or one may use *Tian Wang Bu Xin Dan* (Heavenly Emperor Supplement the Heart Elixir) to calm the heart and quiet the spirit, supplement the kidneys and control fire. If dizziness and tinnitus are severe, add Fructus Lycii Chinensis (*Gou Qi Zi*), Fructus Corni Officinalis (*Shan Zhu Yu*), Flos Chrysanthemi Morifolii (*Gan Hua*), and Concha Haliotidis (*Shi Jue Ming*). If booming heat and sweating are severe, add Concha Ostreae (*Mu Li*) and Radix Et Rhizoma Oryzae Glutinosae (*Nuo Dao Gen Xu*).

Kidney Yang Vacuity & Debility

One should warm the kidneys and supplement yang. The formula to use is *You Gui Wan* (Restore the Right [Kidney] Pills) plus Radix Codonopsis Pilosulae (*Dang Shen*), Fructus Psoraleae Corylifoliae (*Bu Gu Zhi*), Rhizoma Curculiginis Orchoidis (*Xian Mao*), and Herba Epimedii (*Xian Ling Pi*).

Kidney Yin & Yang Dual Vacuity

One should supplement both kidney yin and yang, assisted by downbearing fire. The formula to use is *Zuo Gui Wan* (Restore the Left [Kidney] Pills) and *Er Xian Tang* (Two Immortal Decoction).

Heart/Spleen Dual Vacuity

One should supplement and boost the heart and spleen. The formula to use is *Gui Pi Tang* (Restore the Spleen Decoction). If there is simultaneous kidney vacuity, use *Hei Gui Pi Tang* (Black Restore the Spleen Decoction).

Explanation

1. In clinical practice, this disease is mostly due liver/kidney yin vacuity, and liver fire effulgence. As a rule, the main complaints present in the region of the head and face, such as booming heat (*i.e.*, hot flashes) and sweating. The therapeutic effect for these types of symptoms is always good as long as the proper treatment is given in time. However, this condition may relapse or become chronic if inadequate medication has been administered or if the constitution is particularly vacuous. The authors favor greatly supplementing the qi and blood combined with formulas to enrich yin, subdue yang, and restrain the liver. Then the effects of very good.

2. Menopausal women, due to changes in their physiology, often manifest kidney yin and yang vacuity or liver fire effulgence. It is best if family members try as much as possible to calm the victim at the time of

87

emotional outbursts so as to prevent insomnia and other emotional disturbances.

Treatment

1. *Zhi Bai Di Huang Tang:* This formula is basically the same as *Liu Wei Di Huang Wan* discussed in Section Nine of this same chapter with the addition of Rhizoma Anemarrhenae (*Zhi Mu*) and Cortex Phellodendri (*Huang Bai*).

2. *Tian Wang Bu Xin Dan (*from *Shi Yi De Xiao Fang [Generations of Doctors' Effective Formulas]):* Uncooked Radix Rehmanniae (*Sheng Di*), Radix Scrophulariae Ningpoensis (*Xuan Shen*), Radix Codonopsis Pilosulae (*Dang Shen*), Sclerotium Pararadicis Poriae Cocos (*Fu Shen*), Radix Polygalae Tenuifoliae (*Yuan Zhi*), Tuber Asparagi Cochinensis (*Tian Dong*), Tuber Ophiopogonis Japonicae (*Mai Dong*), Rhizoma Acori Graminei (*Chang Pu*), Semen Biotae Orientalis (*Bai Zi Ren*), prepared Semen Zizyphi Spinosae (*Zao Ren*), Radix Platycodi Grandiflori (*Jie Geng*), Radix Salviae Miltiorrhizae (*Dan Shen*), Cortex Eucommiae Ulmoidis (*Du Zhong*), Radix Angelicae Sinensis (*Dang Gui*), Fructus Schizandrae Chinensis (*Wu Wei Zi*), Radix Stemonae (*Bai Bu*)

3. *You Gui Wan:* See Section Ten, same chapter.

4. *Zuo Gui Wan:* See Section Ten, same chapter.

5. *Er Xian Tang* (an empirical formula): Rhizoma Curculiginis Orchoidis (*Xian Mao*, Herba Epimedii (*Xian Ling Pi*), Radix Morindae Officinalis (*Ba Ji Tian*), Rhizoma Anemarrhenae (*Zhi Mu*), Cortex Phellodendri (*Huang Bai*), Radix Angelicae Sinensis (*Dang Gui*)

6. *Gui Pi Tang:* see Section One, same chapter.

7. *Hei Gui Pi Tang:* This is the same formula as *Gui Pi Tang* discussed in Section One of this same chapter plus prepared Radix Rehmanniae (*Shu Di*).

Chapter Five

Abnormal Vaginal Discharge (*Dai Xia*)

The words *dai xia*, below the belt, may mean two different things. In its broadest sense, *dai xia* refers to various gynecological disorders. Each of these disorders manifest below the waist or *dai mai*. For instance, in the chapter titled "Treatise on Hollow Bones" in the *Su Wen (Simple Questions)* there is, "women's conglomerations and gatherings below the belt." The *Jin Gui Yao Lue (Essentials from the Golden Cabinet)* lists 36 diseases under the heading "*dai xia*." In a narrower sense, this term refers to a sticky, slimy substance flowing from inside a woman's vaginal tract which takes its name from the *dai*. Functionally, the *dai mai* governs the *chong*, *ren* and *du* channels. If the *dai mai* loses its restraint and fails to tie these other vessels properly, then abnormal vaginal discharge is produced. Physiological *dai xia* refers to a scanty discharge which is white in color and has no odor nor is accompanied by any other symptoms. This is most often noted at mid-cycle, just before or after menstruation, during pregnancy, or after sex. If the *dai xia* is excessive in amount, is green, yellow, red, or five-colored, has a foul odor, and is accompanied by soreness and weakness of the body and limbs, dizziness and vertigo, or lumbosacral soreness, this is categorized as a pathological manifestation. Clinically, this is called *dai xia bing* or abnormal vaginal discharge disease.

Although not associated with acute symptoms, vaginal discharge resulting from fluids, humors, and blood pouring downward may embarrass the patient all year round and may be associated with vacuity symptoms, such as low back pain, and chronic detriment and consumption. This frequently leads to the arising of menstrual irregularity or affects reproduction. It may even cause miscarriage after conception. In addition, the patient should be on guard against cancerous changes if excessive and watery vaginal discharge lasts a long time after menopause or if the discharge becomes pussy and has a foul odor.

89

In terms of classification, white, red, yellow, black, green, five-colored, white flux (*bai yin*), and white turbidity (*bai zhuo*) varieties of *dai xia* have been categorized by ancient practitioners. Of these, white turbidity refers to a fetid mucous discharge from the urethra caused by infection due to unhygienic sexual activities. In such cases, a burning pain is often felt at first when passing short, astringent urination which is like rice-washing water. This term is the ancient name for turbid strangury and is typically treated the same as turbid strangury. As for white flux, it is analogous to spermatorrhea in males. Its symptoms include vaginal discharge associated with sexual desire or accompanied by erotic dreams. Therefore, it is treated in the same way as spermatorrhea. Five-colored *dai*, as the name implies, refers to a variegated discharge with a fetid and repulsive odor. It is often found in patients with uterine and cervical carcinomas. As for green and black *dai*, they are rarely encountered in clinical practice. Therefore, only the white, yellow, and red varieties of vaginal discharge are focused on below.

Pathophysiologically, abnormal vaginal discharge is closely related to the *dai* and *ren* vessels. The *dai mai* commands restraint and tying, while the *ren mai* controls in charge of the uterus and fetus. If the *dai* vessel loses its restraining and the *ren mai* does not secure, water dampness turbidity to flow downward in the form of vaginal discharge. Causes leading to the *dai mai* and *ren mai* suffering disease include liver depression/spleen vacuity with dampness and turbidity pouring downward. Life activities may be undisciplined and damp toxins may externally invade, leading to the arising of this condition. It may also be due to excessive bedroom affairs causing detriment and damage to the *chong* and *ren*; kidney vacuity/qi vacuity with essence fluids falling downward; damp heat in the liver channel; or yin vacuity with fire. Thus *dai xia* disease has varied causes. Nevertheless, Fu Qing-zhu has said:

> There can be no *dai xia* without a damp condition and all the varieties of *dai* are due to the *dai mai* not being able to restrain and tie. Hence this disease.

Therefore, although there are various types of abnormal vaginal discharge, its disease causes never go beyond dampness and it is always associated with the *dai mai*. In clinical practice, its treatment is based on these relationships.

The treatment of *dai xia* disease differs according to its differentiation into white *dai*, yellow *dai*, and red *dai*. White vaginal discharge (*bai dai*) due to spleen vacuity and dampness turbidity pouring downward is treated by fortifying the spleen and supporting the center. Therefore, one commonly uses Radix Codonopsis Pilosulae (*Dang Shen*), Rhizoma Atractylodis Macrocephalae (*Bai Zhu*), Radix Astragali Membranacei (*Huang Qi*), Radix Angelicae Sinensis (*Dang Gui*), Radix Dioscoreae Oppositae (*Shan Yao*), Semen Dolichoris Lablab (*Bian Dou*), Semen Euryalis Ferocis (*Qian Shi*), Fructus Alpiniae Oxyphyllae (*Yi Zhi Ren*), and Fructus Corni Officinalis (*Shan Zhu Yu*). If abnormal vaginal discharge is enduring and is watery in consistency, treatment should secure and contain. Therefore one can use Ootheca Mantidis (*Sang Piao Xiao*), Stamen Nelumbinis Nuciferae (*Lian Xu*), Fructus Rosae Laevigatae (*Jin Ying Zi*), Os Draconis (*Long Gu*), and Concha Ostreae (*Mu Li*). If wood depression attacks the spleen, correspondingly, one should add coursing the liver medicinals, such as Radix Albus Paeoniae Lactiflorae (*Bai Shao*), Radix Bupleuri (*Chai Hu*), and Rhizoma Cyperi Rotundi (*Xiang Fu*). If there is damp heat *dai xia*, in order to mainly clear and disinhibit damp heat, commonly use Cortex Phellodendri (*Huang Bai*), Rhizoma Anemarrhenae (*Zhi Mu*), Cortex Ailanthi Altissimi (*Chun Gen Pi*), Rhizoma Dioscoreae Hypoglaucae (*Bi Xie*), Sclerotium Rubrum Poriae Cocos (*Chi Ling*), Caulis Akebiae Mutong (*Mu Tong*), rootlets of Radix Glycyrrhizae (*Gan Cao Xiao*), and white Flos Celosiae Cristatae (*Ji Guan Hua*). If there is turbid strangury, add Folium Pyrrosiae (*Shi Wei*), Spora Lygodii (*Hai Jin Sha*), Succinum (*Hu Po*), Talcum (*Hua Shi*), and Dao Chi San (Abduct the Red Powder). If vaginal discharge is colored red, one can use liver-clearing, yin-enriching medicinals, such as Fructus Ligustri Lucidi (*Nu Zhen Zi*), Herba Ecliptae Prostratae (*Han Lian Cao*), blackened Fructus Gardeniae Jasminoidis (*Shan Zhi*), uncooked Radix Rehmanniae (*Sheng Di*), Cacumen Biotae Orientalis (*Ce Bai Ye*), and Rhizoma Imperatae Cylindricae (*Bai Mao Gen*).

As for set formulas, if there is spleen/stomach deficiency detriment, yang qi falling downward, in order to mainly fortify the spleen and stomach and

91

upbear yang qi, one can use *Bu Zhong Yi Qi Tang* (Supplement the Center & Boost the Qi Decoction) and *Xiang Sha Liu Jun Zi Tang* (Saussurea & Amomum Six Gentlemen Decoction). If due to damp phlegm, treatment should dry dampness and transform phlegm, for which Zhu Dan-xi used Pumice (*Hai Fu Shi*), bile-processed Rhizoma Arisaematis (*Dan Xing*), and Cortex Ailanthi Altissimi (*Chun Gen Pi*). If original qi is insufficient, use *Shou Pi Jian* (Long-life Spleen Decoction). If there is spleen/kidney qi vacuity, use *Shi Quan Da Bu Tang* (Ten [Ingredients] Completely & Greatly Supplementing Decoction). If there is liver depression/ spleen vacuity, use Fu Qing-zhu's *Wan Dai Tang* (End Abnormal Vaginal Discharge Decoction). If there is *dai xia* disease at the same time as vaginal itching, other ingredients compatible with the above decoctions should be given separately for external use. These include Fructus Cnidii Monnieri (*She Chuang Zi*), Fructus Zanthoxyli Bungeani (*Chuan Jiao*), Radix Sophorae Flavescentis (*Ku Shen*), Flos Chrysanthemi Indici (*Ye Ju Hua*), and Alum (*Ming Fan*).

Measures for preventing excessive vaginal discharge consist of controlling and disciplining bedroom affairs and paying attention to hygiene, especially during menstruation, pregnancy, and the puerperium. The external genitalia should be kept clean. Public bath tubs should be avoided. For those with tinea pedis, separate wash basin and towels should be strictly segregated so as not to spread infection to the vagina. In addition, the patient should do her best to avoid emotional disturbance by maintaining a good mood. She should also eat little acrid, peppery or cold, raw foods. In addition, in ancient dynasties there were several prohibitions concerning *dai xia* listed in the literature. For example, the *Dan Xi Xin Fa (Dan-xi's Heart Methods)* says, "Phlegm qi *dai xia* — must cease thick flavors." The *Ru Men Shi Qin (Confucian Responsibility to One's Parents)* says:

In *dai xia*, it is not all right to abruptly use harsh, hot drying medicinals. Drying leads to water drying up internally. If internal water is withered, this must necessarily cause vexatious thirst. Vexatious thirst leads to urination being inhibited. Inhibited urination leads to swollen feet and puffy face. Therefore, soaking results, not treatment.

Both of these above quotations are the valuable experience of our ancestors and are recorded here for our reader's reference.

Section One

White Vaginal Discharge (*Bai Dai*)

If women have a white, sticky, slimy fluid discharge from inside their vagina whose amount is excessive and which is continuous and does not stop by itself, this type of condition is called *bai dai* or white vaginal discharge. *Bai dai* is the most commonly encountered type *dai xia*. Those with this condition often also experience low back soreness, lack of strength, and irregular menstruation. If timely treatment is given for *bai dai* disease, it will do much good for the woman's constitution and will diminish menstrual irregularity, eventually returning it to normal.

Disease Causes, Disease Mechanisms

There is a great deal of discussion in the ancient literature on the origin of this condition. Liao Zhong-chung thought that spleen vacuity, liver depression, and damp earth falling downward are responsible. Zhu Dan-xi thought it was due to phlegm damp pouring downward. Liu He-jian and Zhang Zi-he advanced the theory that it is due to damp heat. Based on these various theories of different schools of medicine combined with its clinical manifestations, the production of this disease is related to spleen vacuity, kidney vacuity, phlegm dampness, and damp heat. Spleen vacuity leads to the finest essence of water and grains not being transported so as to be engendered into blood. Thus it gathers and forms into dampness. This flows to the lower burner, damaging the *ren mai*. The *dai mai* loses its restraint and hence *dai xia* is produced. The kidneys govern sealing and treasuring. If the kidneys are vacuous, sealing and treasuring lose their duty. Essence fluid slips and deserts, therefore becoming *dai xia*. During menstruation, pregnancy, and postpartum, if utensils used are not decontaminated, damp evils may invade from the outside, causing detriment to the *dai* and *ren* and hence *dai xia* is produced.

93

Disease Patterns

Kidney Vacuity

There is excessive vaginal discharge which is clear in color and watery in consistency or like silvery threads. There is also severe low back pain, bilateral pain of the knees, a cold body and chilled limbs, possible insidious pain of the navel and abdomen which is relieved somewhat by obtaining warmth, a possible chilly sensation in the lower abdomen, a deep, fine, forceless pulse, and a pale tongue with a thin, white, moist coating.

Spleen Vacuity

There is excessive vaginal discharge which is white in color or pale yellow, similar to saliva or drool, and which is continues without ceasing. There is also poor eating and drinking, a sallow yellow facial complexion, lack of strength in the four limbs, superficial edema of the face and limbs, lower and upper back soreness and suffering, loose stools, a fine, relaxed (*i.e.*, retarded) pulse, and a pale, fat tongue with a thin, white coating.

Phlegm Dampness

Women with this type of vaginal discharge are usually obese. There is a white vaginal discharge which is thick and sticky, excessive phlegm, nausea, abdominal distention and fatigue after eating. The pulse is fine and slippery and the tongue coating is white and slimy.

Damp Heat

Abnormal vaginal discharge is colored white or a grayish yellow and is thick and sticky in consistency. It may also be either foamy, like tofu, or like curdled milk. If severe, it has a foul odor. Examination of the white discharge reveals the presence of trichomonas or hemophilus infection. There is itching of the external genitalia or burning heat in the vaginal tract. The urination may be short, red, frequent, and numerous. The pulse is slippery and rapid, and the tongue coating is white and slimy.

Treatment

Kidney Vacuity

One should mainly supplement the kidneys and stop *dai*. The formula to use is *Shou Wu Gou Qi Tang* (Polygonum Multiflorum & Lycium Decoction). If kidney vacuity has simultaneous fire effulgence, in order to first clear fire, one can use *Qing Xin Lian Zi Yin* (Clear the Heart Lotus Seed Drink) or *Zhi Zhi Gu Jian Wan* (Straight Finger Secure the Essence Pills). If due to excessive bedroom affairs with slippery discharge not secure, one can use *Jin Suo Si Xian Dan* (Golden Lock Thinking Immortal Elixir) or *Mi Yuan Jian* (Secret Origin Decoction). If kidney vacuity has simultaneous cold, one can use *Nei Bu Wan* (Internally Supplementing Pills). Other ready made (*i.e.*, patent) medicines, such as *Wu Ji Bai Feng Wan* (Black Cock/White Phoenix Pills) and *Zhi Dai Wan* (Stop Abnormal Vaginal Discharge Pills) can also be administered.

Spleen Vacuity

One should fortify the spleen and disinhibit dampness. The formula to use is *Wan Dai Tang* (End Abnormal Vaginal Discharge Decoction). If qi vacuity falls downward, one can use *Bu Zhong Yi Qi Tang* (Supplement the Center & Boost the Qi Decoction).

Phlegm Dampness

One should eliminate dampness and transform phlegm. The formula to use is *Wei Ling Tang* (Stomach *Ling* Decoction). If there is fatness and obesity, one can use *Cang Zhu Chu Pi Wan* (Atractylodes & Ailanthus Pills).

Damp Heat

One should clear and disinhibit damp heat. The formula to use is *Qing Bai San* (Clear the White Powder). If the person is obese with excessive phlegm, add Rhizoma Atractylodis Macrocephalae (*Bai Zhu*) and Rhizoma

Pinelliae Ternatae (*Ban Xia*). If there is red *dai*, add wine stir-fried Radix Scutellariae Baicalensis (*Huang Qin*) and Herba Seu Flos Schizonepetae Tenuifoliae (*Jing Jie*). If there is enduring descent, add prepared Radix Rehmanniae (*Shu Di*) and Concha Ostreae (*Mu Li*). For qi vacuity, add Radix Panacis Ginseng (*Ren Shen*) and Radix Astragali Membranacei (*Huang Qi*). And for low back and knee soreness and pain, add Gelatinum Cornu Cervi (*Lu Jiao Jiao*). If damp heat is exuberant and the body is not vacuous, one can use *Long Dan Xie Gan Tang* (Gentiana Drain the Liver Decoction). One can also use *Er Miao Wan* (Two Miracles Pills) or *San Miao Wan* (Three Miracles Pills) combined with other medicinals decocted for use as an external wash.

Explanation

Women's white vaginal discharge disease is related to undisciplined bedroom affairs and lack of good hygiene. Therefore, those with this disease should live a well-regulated lifestyle and practice good hygiene. In terms of food and drink, she should eat as little as possible of raw, cold, and fatty, slimy foods so as to prevent hindrance to the spleen and stomach's transportation and transmission and thus obstructing the engenderment of damp turbidity. If a post-menopausal woman has excessive, clear, watery white vaginal discharge, a timely gynecological check-up is highly necessary so as to prevent cancerous changes. Wang Meng-ying, a famous practitioner of the Qing Dynasty, once said:

> Women are born with *dai xia*. These fluids are common with the moist root. They are not a disease.

There is another folk saying that, "Ten women, nine have *dai xia*." Nevertheless, if *dai xia* is excessive in amount and there is a yellow face, low back soreness, lack of strength, and, if severe, menstrual irregularity, it must be treated in a timely manner. In that case, it is not appropriate to say, "Women are born with *dai xia* and all have it."

Young girls, adult women, and menopausal women may all be afflicted by *bai dai* disease, and treatment should be given mainly on the basis of an individual discrimination of patterns. However, as a rule, in young girls, this is mostly due to spleen vacuity or external invasion of damp evils. In that case, the doctor should instruct their patient to pay more attention to keeping her external genitalia clean rather than emphasizing medication. In the treatment of senile white vaginal discharge disease, the condition of the spleen and kidneys should be taken into account. Drying dampness medicinals are not appropriate for excessive or prolonged use.

Appended Formulas

1. *Shou Wu Gou Qi Tang (*from *Bing Yu Tang Yan Fang [Proven Formulas from the Crystal Jade Hall]):* Processed Radix Polygoni Multiflori (*Shou Wu*), Fructus Lycii Chinensis (*Gou Qi Zi*), Semen Cuscutae (*Tu Si Zi*), Ootheca Mantidis (*Sang Piao Xiao*), Hallyositum Rubrum (*Chi Shi Zhi*), Rhizoma Cibotii Barometz (*Gou Ji*), stir-fried Cortex Eucommiae Ulmoidis (*Du Zhong*), prepared Radix Rehmanniae (*Shu Di*), Herba Agastachis Seu Pogostemi (*Huo Xiang*), Fructus Amomi (*Sha Ren*)

2. *Qing Xin Lian Zi Yin (*from Tai Ping Hui Min He Ji Ju Fang [Tai Ping Imperial Grace Formulary]): Radix Scutellariae Baicalensis (*Huang Qin*), Tuber Ophiopogonis Japonicae (*Mai Dong*), Cortex Radicis Lycii Chinensis (*Di Gu Pi*), Semen Plantaginis (*Che Qian Zi*), Radix Codonopsis Pilosulae (*Dang Shen*), Radix Astragali Membranacei (*Huang Qi*), Semen Caesalpiniae, Radix Bupleuri (*Chai Hu*), Sclerotium Poriae Cocos, and Radix Glycyrrhizae (*Gan Cao*).

3. *Zhi Zhi Gu Jing Wan (*from *Shen Shi Zun Sheng Shu [Master Shen's Writings on Respecting Life]):* Wine stir-fried Cortex Phellodendri (*Huang Bai*), wine stir-fried Rhizoma Anemarrhenae (*Zhi Mu*), calcined Concha Ostreae (*Mu Li*), calcined Os Draconis (*Long Gu*), Plumula Nelumbinis Nuciferae (*Lian Xin*), Semen Euryalis Ferocis (*Qian Shi*), Fructus Corni Officinalis (*Shan Zhu Yu*), Radix Polygalae Tenuifoliae (*Yuan Zhi*), Sclerotium Rubrum Poriae Cocos (*Chi Fu Ling*)

4. *Jin Suo Si Xian Dan (*from *Shen Shi Zun Sheng Shu [Master Shen's Writings on Respecting Life]):* Plumula Nelumbinis Nuciferae (*Lian Xin*),

97

Semen Euryalis Ferocis (*Qian Shi*), Semen Nelumbinis Nuciferae (*Shi Lian Rou*), Pasta Concentrata Rosae Laevigatae (*Jin Ying Gao*)

5. *Mi Yuan Jian* (from *Jing Yue Quan Shu [Jing-yue's Complete Writings]*): Stir-fried Radix Polygalae Tenuifoliae (*Yuan Zhi*), stir-fried Radix Dioscoreae Oppositae (*Shan Yao*), Semen Euryalis Ferocis (*Qian Shi*), Semen Zizyphi Spinosae (*Zao Ren*), stir-fried Rhizoma Atractylodis Macrocephalae (*Bai Zhu*), Sclerotium Poriae Cocos (*Fu Ling*), Radix Panacis Ginseng (*Ren Shen*), Northern Fructus Schizandrae Chinensis (*Bei Wu Wei Zi*), Fructus Rosae Laevigatae (*Jin Ying Zi*, mix-fried Radix Glycyrrhizae (*Zhi Gan Cao*)

6. *Nei Bu Wan* (from *Nu Ke Qie Yao [Immediate Essentials of Gynecology]*): Cornu Parvum Cervi (*Lu Rong*), Semen Cuscutae (*Tu Si Zi*), Herba Cistanchis (*Rou Cong Rong*), Radix Astragali Membranacei (*Huang Qi*), Cortex Cinnamomi (*Rou Gui*), Ootheca Mantidis (*Sang Piao Xiao*), Semen Astragali Complanati (*Sha Ji Li*), processed Rhizoma Cyperi Rotundi (*Xiang Fu*), Sclerotium Pararadicis Poriae Cocos (*Fu Shen*), Fructus Tribuli Terrestris (*Bai Ji Li*)

7. *Wan Dai Tang* (from *Fu Qing Zhu Nu Ke [Fu Qing-zhu's Gynecology]*): Earth stir-fried Rhizoma Atractylodis Macrocephalae (*Bai Zhu*), stir-fried Radix Dioscoreae Oppositae (*Shan Yao*), Radix Codonopsis Pilosulae (*Dang Shen*), wine stir-fried Radix Albus Paeoniae Lactiflorae (*Bai Shao*), Semen Plantaginis (*Che Qian Zi*), Rhizoma Atractylodis (*Cang Zhu*), Pericarpium Citri Reticulatae (*Chen Pi*), carbonized Herba Seu Flos Schizonepetae Tenuifoliae (*Jing Jie*), Radix Bupleuri (*Chai Hu*), Radix Glycyrrhizae (*Gan Cao*)

8. *Bu Zhong Yi Qi Tang:* See Section One, Chapter Four.

9. *Wei Ling Tang* (from *Zheng Zhi Zhun Sheng [Patterns & Treatments Norms & Criteria]*): Cortex Magnoliae Officinalis (*Chuan Po*), Pericarpium Citri Reticulatae (*Bai Zhu*), Rhizoma Atractylodis (*Cang Zhu*), Rhizoma Atractylodis Macrocephalae (*Bai Zhu*), Sclerotium Poriae Cocos

(*Fu Ling*), Rhizoma Alismatis (*Ze Xie*), Ramulus Cinnamomi (*Gui Zhi*), Sclerotium Polypori Umbellati (*Zhu Ling*), Radix Glycyrrhizae (*Gan Cao*)

10. *Chang Shu Chu Pi Wan:* Rhizoma Atractylodis (*Cang Zhu*), Cortex Ailanthi Altissimi (*Chun Gen Pi*), Rhizoma Arisaematis (*Nan Xing*), Rhizoma Pinelliae Ternatae (*Ban Xia*), Pumice (*Hai Fu Shi*), Radix Ligustici Wallichii (*Chuan Xiong*), Rhizoma Cyperi Rotundi (*Xiang Fu*), blast-fried Rhizoma Zingiberis (*Pao Jiang*). In summer, remove blast-fried Rhizoma Zingiberis and add Talcum (*Hua Shi*). Grind the above ingredients and make into pills with vinegar.

11. *Qing Bai San:* Radix Angelicae Sinensis (*Dang Gui*), Radix Ligustici Wallichii (*Chuan Xiong*), Radix Albus Paeoniae Lactiflorae (*Bai Shao*), uncooked Radix Rehmanniae (*Sheng Di*), saltwater stir-fried Cortex Phellodendri (*Huang Bai*), wine stir-fried Cortex Ailanthi Altissimi (*Chun Gen Pi*), Bulbus Fritillariae (*Bei Mu*), blast-fried carbonized Rhizoma Zingiberis (*Pao Jiang Tan*), Radix Glycyrrhizae (*Gan Cao*)

12. *Long Dan Xie Gan Tang* (from *Lan Shi Mi Cang [Secret Treasury of the Orchid Pavilion]*): Radix Angelicae Sinensis (*Dang Gui*), uncooked Radix Rehmanniae (*Sheng Di*), Rhizoma Alismatis (*Ze Xie*), Fructus Gardeniae Jasminoidis (*Shan Zhi*), Radix Scutellariae Baicalensis (*Huang Qin*), Semen Plantaginis (*Che Qian Zi*), Radix Gentianae Scabrae (*Long Dan Cao*), Radix Bupleuri (*Chai Hu*), Radix Glycyrrhizae (*Gan Cao*)

13. *Er Miao Wan* (from *Dan Xi Xin Fa [Dan-xi's Heart Methods]*): Rhizoma Atractylodis (*Cang Zhu*), Cortex Phellodendri (*Huang Bai*)

14. *San Miao Wan* (from *Dan Xi Xin Fa [Dan-xi's Heart Methods]*): Rhizoma Atractylodis (*Cang Zhu*), Cortex Phellodendri (*Huang Bai*), Radix Achyranthis Bidentatae (*Huai Niu Xi*)

Section Two

Red Vaginal Discharge (*Chi Dai*)

Dai xia which is either colored pale red and is sticky and thick, is fresh red, or looks like or is expelled with blood is called *chi dai*, red abnormal vaginal discharge. If white *dai* has within it red *dai*, this is called red and white *dai* or *chi bai dai*. Clinically, red and white *dai* and red *dai* are generally treated as red *dai*.

Disease Causes, Disease Mechanisms

The origin of red *dai* is due to either damp heat or heart/liver channel depressive fire blazing and exuberance. This then eventually causes deficiency detriment to the yin blood. Fu Qing-zhu says:

The *dai mai* flows freely to the kidneys, and kidney qi flows freely to the liver. If, in women, worry and thinking damage the spleen and if depression and anger damage the liver, this may result in liver channel depressive fire blazing internally. This horizontally checks spleen earth. Spleen earth is then not able to transport and transform. This results in damp heat due to the brewing of qi within the *dai mai*. The liver does not treasure the blood which seeps internally within the *dai mai*. Because the spleen qi has suffered damage, transportation and transformation have no strength. Damp heat qi follows downward falling, with the blood also completely descending. This results in the blood being expelled and the bloody shaped signs. Replete blood and dampness are not able to de divided into two...The treatment method is to clear liver fire and support the spleen qi.

Miao Zhong-chun said:

Red *dai* is mostly due to the two fires of the heart and liver. If this constantly blazes without cease, over time, yin blood becomes gradually vacuous and central qi gradually suffers detriment. Thus there is red *dai*.

100

Therefore, the causes of this disease can not be further differentiated beyond the two—damp heat and blood vacuity. However, whether damp heat is heavy and predominates or whether blood vacuity is heavy and predominates must always be differentiated.

Disease Patterns

Predominant Damp Heat

The abnormal vaginal discharge is colored red, is sticky and turbid, and has a foul odor. It dribbles and drips without ceasing. Occasionally it is mixed with a whitish vaginal discharge. If heat is severe, there is oral thirst, a bitter taste in the mouth, and reddish urine. The tongue is red with a thick, slimy or yellow coating, and the pulse is mostly slippery and rapid.

Predominant Blood Vacuity

The abnormal vaginal discharge is red in color or like fresh blood and is scanty in amount. It is thick and sticky and has a foul odor. There is heart vexation, oral thirst, burning heat in the hands, feet, and heart, dry stools, and a fine, rapid or vacuous rapid pulse if blood vacuity produces heat. There is chest and lateral costal fullness, oppression, and vexation, emotional depression and lack of relaxation, and a wiry, rapid pulse image, if there is blood vacuity and liver depression. If red *dai* endures for a long time and does not stop and if there is essence spirit fatigue, no thought for food and drink, a pale white tongue, and a fine, weak pulse, this is blood vacuity and also qi vacuity.

Treatment

Predominant Damp Heat

One should clear heat and dispel dampness. If heat is mild, the formula to use is *Jia Jian Qing Bao Yin* (Additions & Subtractions Clear the Uterus

101

Drink). If heat is severe, the formula to use is *Long Dan Xie Gan Tang* (Gentiana Drain the Liver Decoction).

Predominant Blood Vacuity

For blood vacuity with internal heat, one should enrich yin and clear heat. The formula to use is *Qin Lian Si Wu Tang* (Scutellaria & Coptis Four Materials Decoction) or *Bao Yin Jian* (Protect the Yin Decoction). For blood vacuity and liver depression, one should nourish the blood and clear fire, rectify the qi and resolve depression. The formula to use is *Miao Xiang San* (Miraculous Fragrant Powder), *Qing Gan Zhi Lin Tang* (Clear the Liver & Stop Strangury Decoction), or a combination of these two remedies with corresponding additions and subtractions. Or one may use *Xiao Chai Hu Tang* (Minor Bupleurum Decoction) plus Rhizoma Coptidis Chinensis (*Huang Lian*) and Fructus Gardeniae Jasminoidis (*Zhi Zi*). For qi vacuity downward falling or qi and blood completely vacuous, use *Bu Zhong Yi Qi Tang* (Supplement the Center & Boost the Qi Decoction) or *Ba Zhen Tang* (Eight Pearls Decoction) in order to supplement and nourish the qi and blood.

Explanation

1. Red vaginal discharge and bloody strangury are not the same. Red *dai* exits from the vaginal tract. Bloody *lin* exists from the urinary tract. Clinically, gynecological examination or urine examination can clearly differentiate these.

2. Red vaginal discharge is by far most often mixed with a whitish vaginal discharge. Hence, this is typically called red and white vaginal discharge. Red vaginal discharge often dribbles downward and is not excessive in amount. If, in clinical practice, it appears greatly excessive, this is mostly due to blood vacuity, with a few cases being due to damp heat. Therefore, physicians in ancient dynasties emphasized the treatment of this disease by primarily treating the blood and clearing the constructive.

102

3. If red *dai* appears mid-cycle in a woman's menstrual cycle, this should be distinguished from mid-cycle bleeding. This may be confirmed by taking the basal body temperature.

4. If red *dai* appears after menopause, the patient should be instructed to seek medical advice so as to prevent possible cancerous changes.

Appended Formulas

1. *Jia Jian Qing Bao Yin:* Cortex Phellodendri (*Huang Bai*), Semen Plantaginis (*Che Qian Zi*), Radix Angelicae Sinensis (*Dang Gui*), stir-fried Radix Albus Paeoniae Lactiflorae (*Bai Shao*), Fructus Gardeniae Jasminoidis (*Shan Zhi*), Sclerotium Poriae Cocos (*Fu Ling*), Cortex Radicis Lycii Chinensis (*Di Gu Pi*), Rhizoma Anemarrhenae (*Zhi Mu*), Pericarpium Citri Reticulatae (*Chen Pi*), stir-fried Radix Scutellariae Baicalensis (*Huang Qin*), Radix Glycyrrhizae (*Gan Cao*)

2. *Long Dan Xie Gan Tang:* See Section One, Chapter Four.

3. *Qin Lian Si Wu Tang:* See Section One, Chapter Four.

4. *Bao Yin Jian (*from *Shen Shi Zhun Sheng Shu [Master Shen's Writings on Respecting Life]):* Uncooked Radix Rehmanniae (*Sheng Di*), prepared Radix Rehmanniae (*Shu Di*), Radix Albus Paeoniae Lactiflorae (*Bai Shao*), Radix Dioscoreae Oppositae (*Shan Yao*), Radix Dipsaci (*Xu Duan*), Cortex Phellodendri (*Huang Bai*), Radix Scutellariae Baicalensis (*Huang Qin*), Radix Glycyrrhizae (*Gan Cao*)

5. *Miao Xiang San (*from *Su Shen Liang Fang [Suzhou Shen's Fine Formulas]):* Radix Codonopsis Pilosulae (*Dang Shen*), Sclerotium Pararadicis Poriae Cocos (*Fu Shen*), Radix Polygalae Tenuifoliae (*Yuan Zhi*), Radix Dioscoreae Oppositae (*Shan Yao*), Radix Astragali Membranacei (*Huang Qi*), Cinnabar (*Zhu Sha*, Radix Saussureae Seu Vladimiriae (*Mu Xiang*), Radix Platycodi Grandiflori (*Jie Geng*), Secretio Moschi Moschiferi (*She Xiang*), Sclerotium Poriae Cocos (*Fu Ling*), Radix

Glycyrrhizae (*Gan Cao*). Grind these ingredients into powder and take 9g per day with warm wine.

6. *Qing Gan Zhi Lin Tang (*from *Fu Qing Zhu Nu Ke [Fu Qing-zhu's Gynecology]): Cortex Radicis Moutan (*Dan Pi*), Cortex Phellodendri (*Huang Bai*), Radix Achyranthis Bidentatae (*Niu Xi*), stir-fried Radix Albus Paeoniae Lactiflorae (*Bai Shao*), Radix Angelicae Sinensis (*Dang Gui*), uncooked Radix Rehmanniae (*Sheng Di*), Gelatinum Corii Asini (*E Jiao*), wine stir-fried Rhizoma Cyperi Rotundi (*Xiang Fu*), Semen Glycinis Hispidae (*Xiao Hei Dou*), Fructus Zizyphi Jujubae (*Hong Zao*)

7. *Xiao Chai Hu Tang (*from *Shang Han Lun [Treatise on Damage Due to Cold]): Radix Bupleuri (*Chai Hu*), Radix Scutellariae Baicalensis (*Huang Qin*), Radix Codonopsis Pilosulae (*Dang Shen*), processed Rhizoma Pinelliae Ternatae (*Ban Xia*), mix-fried Radix Glycyrrhizae (*Zhi Gan Cao*), uncooked Rhizoma Zingiberis (*Sheng Jiang*), Fructus Zizyphi Jujubae (*Da Zao*)

8. *Bu Zhong Yi Qi Tang:* See Section One, Chapter Four.

9. *Ba Zhen Tang (*from *Zheng Zhi Zhun Sheng [Patterns & Treatments Norms & Criteria): Radix Codonopsis Pilosulae (*Dang Shen*), Sclerotium Poriae Cocos (*Fu Ling*), Rhizoma Atractylodis Macrocephalae (*Bai Zhu*), mix-fried Radix Glycyrrhizae (*Zhi Gan Cao*), Radix Ligustici Wallichii (*Chuan Xiong*), Radix Angelicae Sinensis (*Dang Gui*), Radix Albus Paeoniae Lactiflorae (*Bai Shao*), prepared Radix Rehmanniae (*Shu Di*)

Section Three

Yellow Vaginal Discharge (*Huang Dai*)

If a woman's *dai xia* is colored yellow, is sticky and slimy, and has a foul odor, this is called yellow vaginal discharge or *huang dai*. In the Jin

Dynasty, yellow *dai* was called yellow flooding (*huang beng*). The *Mai Jing (Pulse Classic)* says, "*Huang beng* resembles in form a rotten melon." The *Zhu Bing Yuan Hou Lun (Treatise on the Origin & Symptoms of Various Diseases)* is where this condition is first referred to as yellow *dai*.

Disease Causes, Disease Mechanisms

Yellow *dai* is mostly due to spleen earth damp exuberance which leads to its arising. If the spleen is not fortified and does not transport, water dampness brews and binds. If this endures, this brewing leads to transformative heat. Damp heat evils invade the *ren mai* and the *dai mai* loses its restraint. This then produces yellow *dai*. Yellow *dai* disease is categorized as spleen channel damp depression. However, within spleen dampness there is spleen dampness/liver heat and spleen vacuity with dampness which are not the same. Their clinical manifestations and their treatment principles, formulas, and methods are also not the same.

Disease Patterns

Spleen Dampness/Liver Heat

The abnormal vaginal discharge is colored yellow, fresh and bright like pus, or it may look like a rotten melon or strong tea. Its odor is foul. The area of the genitals is swollen, painful, itching, or burning hot and not soothed. Urination is astringent and painful or frequent and numerous, short and scanty. The tongue is red and its coating is thin and yellow or yellow and slimy. The pulse is wiry and rapid or slippery and rapid.

Spleen Vacuity Mixed with Dampness

The abnormal vaginal discharge is colored pale yellow, its amount is excessive, it dribbles and drips without cease, and its foul odor is mild and scanty. There is spiritual fatigue, a liking for sleep, weakness of the four limbs, fatigue after eating, abdominal distention, clear, long urination, a pale tongue with a thin, white coating, and a soggy, fine pulse.

105

Treatment

Spleen Dampness/Liver Heat

One should mainly support the spleen, dispel dampness, and clear heat. the formula to use is *Yi Huang Tang* (Change Yellow Decoction) or *Qin Zhu Chu Pi Wan* (Scutellaria, Atractylodes & Cortex Ailanthi Pills).

Spleen Vacuity Mixed with Dampness

One should fortify the spleen, boost the qi, and transform dampness. The formula to use is *Xiang Sha Liu Jun Zi Tang* (Saussurea & Amomum Six Gentlemen Decoction). If there is spiritual fatigue and weak limbs, a sagging downward feeling in the lower abdomen, and low back soreness with *dai xia* which dribbles and drips without cease, one can use *Bu Zhong Yi Qi Tang* (Supplement the Center & Boost the Qi Decoction).

Explanation

1. If, in *dai xia* disease, there is itching of the external genitalia, one can also use externally *Xun Xi Fang* (Steaming & Washing Formula): Fructus Cnidii Monnieri (*She Chuang Zi*, Radix Sophorae Flavescentis (*Ku Shen*), Flos Chrysanthemi Indici (*Ye Ju Hua*), Fructus Zanthoxyli Bungeani (*Chuan Jiao*), Alum (*Ming Fan*). Each day 1 *ji*. Decoct in water and discard the dregs. Steam the external genitalia with this medicinal juice. After it has cooled, use it as a sitz bath, 1-2 times per day, washing for 3-5 days. Stop washing during the menstruation.

2. Timely gynecological examination is highly recommended not only for those whose abnormal vaginal discharge is mixed with variegated colors with a bad odor but also for those with abdominal pain and irregular menstruation, and especially for those after menopause with the purpose of excluding the suspicion of malignant tumor of the urogenital system.

3. If there is *dai xia* disease due to damp heat or internal obstruction by damp toxins, treatment at first should not necessarily consist of stopping

dai. This may result in the retention of damp turbid evils and give rise to abdominal distention and pain. Only when the vaginal discharge turns white or watery is it all right to secure, astringe, and stop *dai.*

Appended Formulas

1. *Yi Huang Tang (*from *Fu Qing Zhu Nu Ke (Fu Qing-zhu's Gynecology):* Stir-fried Radix Dioscoreae Oppositae, stir-fried Semen Euryalis Ferocis (*Qian Shi*), saltwater stir-fried Cortex Phellodendri (*Huang Bai*), wine stir-fried Semen Plantaginis (*Che Qian Zi*), Semen Ginkgonis Bilobae (*Bai Guo*), 10 pieces, smashed

2. *Qin Zhu Chu Pi Wan (*from *Shen Shi Zun Sheng Shu [Master Shen's Writings on Respecting Life]):* Radix Scutellariae Baicalensis (*Huang Qin*), Rhizoma Atractylodis Macrocephalae (*Bai Zhu*), Cortex Ailanthi Altissimi (*Chun Gen Pi*), Radix Albus Paeoniae Lactiflorae (*Bai Shao*), Fructus Corni Officinalis (*Shan Zhu Yu*), Radix Angelicae Sinensis (*Dang Gui*), Rhizoma Coptidis Chinensis (*Huang Lian*)

3. *Bu Zhong Yi Qi Tang:* See Section One, Chapter Four.

4. *Xiang Sha Liu Jun Zi Tang:* See Section Two, Chapter Four.

Chapter Six

Gestational Disorders (*Tai Qian Bing*)

Tai qian bing (literally before birth diseases) refer to any disorder taking place during the period from conception to delivery. The most commonly encountered disorders during gestation are vomiting during pregnancy, abdominal pain, fetal stirring restlessness, fetal leakage precipitating blood, falling fetus, slippery fetus, swelling and distention, fetal epilepsy, and rotated uterus. These conditions often endanger the lives of the mother and fetus. Therefore, practitioners of past ages all regarded gestational diseases as one of the main chapters in the specialty of gynecology. However, before proceeding to the specific treatments of each gestational disease, some essential points on the principals of diagnosis, lifestyle, and medicinal prohibitions during pregnancy are introduced below.

1. Diagnosing Pregnancy

The early diagnosis of pregnancy is of clinical importance in order to avoid any harmful influences which might affect the body or which might cause bleeding and miscarriage. The diagnosis of early pregnancy in TCM is made by means of observation, interrogation, auscultation/olfaction, and palpation.

Observation

The facial complexion typically looks like the normal person's or it may be slightly sallow and yellow or grayish white. There is fatigue and lack of strength and occasional desire to sit and lie down. After the second month of pregnancy, the breasts are enlarged and the nipples and areola have darkened in color. Often the area around the nipple is dotted with tiny nodules. the tongue has a thin, white coating or may be sticky and slimy.

Interrogation

A) Questioning concerning menstruation:

Married women of child-bearing age with otherwise regular cycles should be suspected of being pregnant if their periods are 10 days overdue. The longer the delay, the more suspicion should arise. Cessation of menstruation is the earliest and most important signal of conception, even though a number of women whose periods are interrupted may not have conceived. Diagnosis can be made only with reference to other signs and symptoms. However, some women may become pregnant even while breast-feeding and a few women may still menstruate regularly for the first 4-5 months after conception but with reduced volume.

B) Questioning concerning accompanying symptoms:

In the early stages of pregnancy, there may be various degrees of nausea and vomiting and are most likely to occur in the early morning. Increased secretion of saliva, lack of appetite, preference for certain foods and dislike of oily, slimy foods, or a certain specific smell may develop. In addition, weakness of the four limbs, somnolence, dizziness, spiritual fatigue, a cold body, or breast distention may all be noticed. These conditions usually subside after 3-4 months. However, these responses to pregnancy may vary greatly in severity and duration from case to case depending upon the body's strength or weakness, past reproductive history, and individual differences in mental and physical labor. Clinical experience so far suggests that those who are in good health, are multiparas, and who do physical labor are typically affected by these conditions less severely and for a shorter period of time. There are exceptional cases where women feel just as normal as usual. If the body is weak, if there are typically many diseases, if the woman is a primipara, and she does mostly mental work, these conditions are often more severe and last for a longer period of time.

Auscultation/Olfaction

Nothing (of significance) can be detected from this procedure since pregnancy is a normal physiological phenomenon.

Palpation

At the being of pregnancy, yin and yang congeal and unite and the fetal origin binds at that time. Typically, the pulse of pregnancy at the *guan* and *chi* positions are rapid and slippery. Although individuals may differ, still they are not other than slippery, uninhibited, harmonious, and level.

Besides observation, interrogation, auscultation/olfaction, and palpation, pelvic examination, urine testing, assessment of the basal temperature, and other such methods may be simultaneously employed in order to confirm pregnancy as early as possible.

2. Lifestyle During Pregnancy

It is known to all that adequate attention paid to life style during pregnancy is very important not only for preventing possible abnormalities before, during, and after delivery but also for assuring the safety and health of the mother and the newborn. Fetal education as put forth by the ancients is meaningful. As far back as the Southern & Northern Period, Xue Zi-chai, a famous physician of his time, advanced the theory of a nourishing the fetus method for each month. In the Tang Dynasty, the *Qian Jin Yao Fang (Prescriptions [Worth a] Thousand [Pieces of] Gold)* also contained principles and methods for nourishing the fetus in each of the 10 months.

In the *Bian Chan Xu He (Ensuring a Harmonious Delivery)* there is the following quotation regarding the essentials of hygiene (literally, defending life) for pregnant women:

> Avoid the random use of medicinals, the excessive drinking of wine, and reckless acupuncture and moxibustion...do not wear clothes which make one too warm and do not eat till too full. If the spleen and stomach are not harmonious, the constructive and defensive will be vacuous and cowardly, and this must necessarily result in many diseases.

In summarizing the experience of practitioners of past ages, the following points can be generalized: 1) It is essential that the essence spirit remain optimistic. 2) It is essential that food and drink be easily digestible and nutritious. One should not overeat acrid, peppery stuffs. 3) One should refrain from overtaxation or excessive leisure. It is essential that they get exercise and sufficient sleep. One should keep their urination and defecation open and smoothly flowing. One should not tie strings or belts around their body too tightly. Nor should they take medicine at random. Furthermore, they should not receive reckless acupuncture and moxibustion, not lift heavy objects, and not engage in bedroom affairs.

3. Medicinals Prohibited from Use During Pregnancy

The ancients had 3 prohibitions during pregnancy. The first prohibition was against diaphoresis. Forcing excessive sweat looses yang and this damages the qi. The second prohibition is against precipitation. Forcing excessive precipitations looses yin and this damages the blood. The third prohibition is against disinhibiting urination. Forcing excessive urination damages the fluids and humors. In addition, in the *Ji Yin Gang Mu (Detailed Outline of Yin)*, *Yi Xue Xin Wu (Heart Awakening in the Study of Medicine)*, *Fu Ren Da Quan Liang Fine (A Great, Complete [Collection] of Fine Formulas for Women)*, *Bian Chan Xu He (Ensuring a Harmonious Delivery)*, and other such medical texts, there are verses concerning prohibitions during pregnancy which are well written and are widely popular. The following is an example of a list of prohibited medicinals found in *Bian Chan Xu He (Ensuring a Harmonious Delivery)*:

Hirudo (*Shui Zhi*) and Tabanus (*Meng Chong*) are prohibited during pregnancy as are the combination of Radix Aconiti (*Wu Tou*) and Radix Lateralis Praeparatus Aconiti Carmichaeli (*Fu Zi*). The combination of Radix Puerariae (*Ge Gen*), Mercury (*Shu Ying*), and Semen Crotonis Tiglii (*Ba Dou*); the combination of Radix Achyranthis Bidentatae (*Niu Xi*), Semen Coicis Lachryma-jobi (*Yi Mi*), and Scolopendra Subspinipes (*Wu Gong*); the combination of Rhizoma Sparganii (*San Leng*), Haematitum (*Dai Zhe*, and Flos Daphnis Genkwae (*Xuan Hua*); the combination of Radix Euphorbiae Seu Knoxiae (*Da Ji*), Periostracum Serpentis (*She Tui*), Orpiment (*Huang Ci*), and Realgar (*Xiong*); the combination of Mirabilitum (*Mang Xiao*), Cortex Radicis Moutan (*Dan Pi*), Cortex Cinnamomi (*Gui*), Flos Immaturus Sophorae Japonicae (*Huai Hua*), Cornu Rhinocerotis (*Xi Jiao*), and Fructus Gleditschiae Chinensis (*Zao Jiao*); the combination of Rhizoma Pinelliae Ternatae (*Ban Xia*), Rhizoma Arisaematis (*Nan Xing*), and Medulla Tetrapanacis Papyriferi (*Tong Cao*); the combination of Herba Dianthi (*Qu Mai*), dry Rhizoma Zingiberis (*Gan Jiang*), Semen Pruni Persicae (*Tao Ren*), Sal Ammoniac (*Nao Sha*), Resina Rhi Vernicifluae (*Gan Qi*), and Crab Claw (*Xie Jiao Jia*); the combination of Tuber Tinosporae Caillipis (*Di Dan*) and Rhizoma Imperatae Cylindricae (*Mao Gen*).

In addition, any ingredient with similar properties to that of the foregoing list should also be included amongst these prohibitions.

From the above passages describing the 3 prohibitions and prohibited medicinals during pregnancy, we can see how discriminating earlier people were regarding medication for expectant mothers. However, appropriate symptomatic dosage (with otherwise contraindicated ingredients) should be given without hesitation if the ingredients are considered necessary to correct critical conditions. This is what is called "medication speared at the disease." It should be immediately ceased as soon as the disease has diminished. The dosages of such ingredients prescribed during pregnancy are often more carefully weighed, especially for those pregnant women whose body is vacuous or whose lower origin is not secure or those with habitual miscarriage. Therefore, in the treatment of the typical diseases of pregnant women, one should try to avoid the use of these medicinals when possible.

113

Section One

Nausea &Vomiting (*E Zu*)

Nausea and vomiting are commonly seen diseases during early pregnancy. Their main symptoms are nausea, vomiting, depressed appetite, picky appetite, and a desire for sour and salty foods.

Disease Causes, Disease Mechanisms

The *Jin Gui Yao Lue (Essentials from the Golden Cabinet)* says that nausea and vomiting during pregnancy involves the two channels of the liver and spleen and mainly the spleen and stomach. The causes of nausea and vomiting are:

Upward Counterflow of Liver Qi

After conception, the menstruation ceases and stops. The visceral qi is thus not diffused. The liver qi becomes tense and counterflows upward.

Upward Surging of Stomach Fire

This is due to most pregnant women having internal heat. If stomach fire's root is exuberant, after conception, heat will congest in the stomach. This leads to the arising of nausea and vomiting.

Yin Vacuity, Floating Yang

As the fetal origin initially binds, true yin congeals and gathers below. If the pregnant woman's kidney yin is insufficient, it is not capable of performing above. Thus vacuous yang floats upward and this results in nausea and vomiting.

114

Spleen/Stomach Vacuity Weakness

Pregnant women are commonly associated with spleen/stomach vacuity. Their digestion is not strong, and the central qi is vacuous and weak. Phlegm rheum stops and binds and food and drink stop and stagnate. Or the spleen and stomach may be vacuous and cold. This is able to lead to the arising of nausea and vomiting.

Disease Patterns

Upward Counterflow of Liver Qi

Eating leads to vomiting of the food eaten and drinking leads to vomiting of water. There is oppression within the heart, belching, a dry mouth and parched tongue, picky appetite, aversion to food, desire for sour foods, dizziness, vertigo, and essence spirit fatigue. The four limbs are sluggish and there is desire to sleep. The tongue coating is thick and slimy, and the pulse image is wiry and slippery or flowing and uninhibited.

Upward Surging of Stomach Fire

Commonly there is a dry mouth and parched throat, red eyes, red face, gum swelling and pain, vexatious heat within the heart, and thirst with a desire for chilled drinks but drinking induces vomiting. The stools are constipated and the urination is short and red. The tongue is red or has a scanty coating. The pulse image is wiry and rapid.

Yin Vacuity, Floating Yang

There is dizziness, tinnitus, heart palpitations, loss of sleep, vexatious heat in the five hearts, dry mouth, and thinking of drinking. After eating, there is vomiting. The tongue is read, and if, severe, there is no coating. The pulse image is vacuous and weak or fine and rapid.

Spleen/Stomach Vacuity Weakness

There is phlegm and food stopped and stagnant, diminished eating and drinking, nausea at the smell of food, and possible acid eructations. Phlegm drool congests and is exuberant, and vomiting does not stop. The tongue is pale or fat and has a white, slimy coating. The pulse image is wiry and slippery.

Treatment

Upward Counterflow of Liver Qi

One should normalize the flow of the liver and downbear counterflow, fortify the spleen and boost the qi. The formula to use is *Shun Gan Yi Qi Tang* (Normalize the Liver & Boost the Qi Decoction) or *Ren Shen Ju Pi Tang* (Ginseng & Orange Peel Decoction).

Upward Surging of Stomach Fire

One should clear heat and settle vomiting. The formula to use is *Jia Wei Wen Dan Tang* (Added Flavors Warm the Gallbladder Decoction).

Yin Vacuity, Floating Yang

One should boost the kidneys and subdue yang, enrich yin and downbear counterflow. The formula to use is *Zhi Bai Di Huang Wan* (Anemarrhena & Phellodendron Rehmannia Pills) given as a decoction plus Os Draconis (*Long Gu*), Concha Ostreae (*Mu Li*), Caulis In Taeniis Bambusae (*Zhu Ru*), and uncooked Rhizoma Zingiberis (*Sheng Jiang*). Or one can use *Zi Yin Jiang Ni Tang* (Enrich Yin & Downbear Counterflow Decoction) if there are heart palpitations and insomnia plus Semen Biotae Orientalis (*Bai Zi Ren*), stir-fried Semen Zizyphi Spinosae (*Zao Ren*), or Caulis Polygoni Multiflori (*Ye Jiao Teng*).

Spleen/Stomach Vacuity Weakness

One should fortify the spleen and boost the qi, harmonize the stomach and settle vomiting. The formula to use is *Zhu Ru Tang* (Caulis Bambusae Decoction) or *Xiang Sha Liu Jun Zi Tang* (Saussurea & Amomum Six Gentlemen Decoction) and *Er Chen Tang* (Two Aged [Ingredients] Decoction).

Explanation

1. Most women in the early stage of pregnancy most have depressed appetite and symptoms of nausea and vomiting . These may be either light or heavy. If mild, one does not have to administer medicinals. Frequent, light meals or eating whatever is desired will help relieve the problem. However, if vomiting will not stop, one should respond with timely treatment. Otherwise, the health of both the mother and child may be jeopardized, since severe vomiting without cure may lead to emaciation, malnutrition, dehydration, and, if severe, even miscarriage. In addition to Chinese medicinals, intravenous transfusion may also be employed. In some cases, a medicinal soup made from stir-fried polished rice can be taken for a month instead of medicinals whenever medicinals fail to have any effect. In the Ming Dynasty, Lou Quan-shan said:

> One can use *Chao Geng Mi Tang* (Stir-fried Polished Rice Soup) drunk as a tea and stop medicinals. In one month, there will be spontaneous cure.

The patient is also advised to try another technique called the fragrant opening vapor method. This consists of boiling a handful of fresh Herba Coriandri Sativi (*Yan Sui*, also called *Xiang Cai*) together with 3g each of Folium Perillae Frutescentis (*Su Ye*) and Herba Agastachis Seu Pogostemi (*Huo Xiang*) and 6g of Pericarpium Citri Reticulatae (*Chen Pi*) and Fructus Amomi (*Sha Ren*). The patient is instructed to inhale this medicinal vapor puffed out from the spout of a kettle. This vapor has the function of broadening the chest and levelling counterflow, delighting the spleen and

117

rousing the stomach. Following this, the patient may take a little, easily digestible food.

2. In clinical practice, this disease is mostly due to liver effulgence, spleen/stomach vacuity weakness, and phlegm dampness obstructing and stagnating. Commonly used formulas are *Fu Ling Ban Xia Tang* (Poria & Pinellia Decoction) and *Shun Gan Yi Qi Tang* (Normalize the Liver & Boost the Qi Decoction). *Shun Gan Yi Qi Tang* has the functions of levelling the liver and fortifying the spleen, normalizing the flow of qi and transforming phlegm. Therefore, it can be employed with additions and subtractions in the treatment of morning sickness of various etiologies. Because the original formula of *Shun Gan Yi Qi Tang* contains prepared Radix Rehmanniae (*Shu Di*) which is greatly slimy and Fructus Perillae Frutescentis (*Su Zi*) which is oily, these can be removed and add ginger(-processed) Rhizoma Pinelliae Ternatae (*Ban Xia*). If there is chest oppression, add Caulis Perillae Frutescentis (*Su Gen*), Herba Agastachis Seu Pogostemi (*Huo Xiang*), and Fructus Cardamomi (*Kou Ren*). If vomiting is severe, add Terra Flava Usta (*Fu Long Gan*). If the body is cold, add uncooked Rhizoma Zingiberis (*Sheng Jiang*) and Caulis Perillae Frutescentis (*Su Gen*). If there is lateral costal pain, add Radix Bupleuri (*Chai Hu*). If there is headache, add Concha Haliotidis (*Shi Jue Ming*). If there is constipation, remove Rhizoma Atractylodis Macrocephalae (*Bai Zhu*) and add Fructus Trichosanthis Kirlowii (*Quan Gua Lou*). If there is low back soreness, add Ramus Loranthis Seu Visci (*Sang Ji Sheng*) and Cortex Eucommiae Ulmoidis (*Du Zhong*). Following the pattern, add and subtract correspondingly.

3. Rhizoma Pinelliae Ternatae (*Ban Xia*) was one of the originally prohibited medicinals during pregnancy. However, Pinellia once it has been processed is a very effective medicinal for stopping vomiting and it is therefore commonly used in clinical practice. It has no bad side effects, and one can use it with one's mind at ease. Terra Flava Usta (*Fu Long Gan*), also called *Zao Xin Tu*, is also an effective medicinal for severe vomiting in pregnancy. As much as 30g can be used per dose.

118

4. Morning sickness in the early stage of pregnancy can be treated with dietary therapy without administering medicinals if mild. Or this may be combined with dietary therapy to disperse and eliminate the symptoms more quickly. Patients are advised to eat their favorite, easily digestible foods in frequent, light meals and never to take any raw, chilled, or oily, slimy foods. Following this, the effects of medicinals will then be good.

5. It is not uncommon to pregnant women with severe vomiting to refuse to take large amounts of bitter-flavored Chinese medicinals. After administration, they may vomit everything back up. One way to cope with this situation is to drink the decoction in several small portions or first rubbing the tongue with a slice of fresh ginger before drinking the decoction. This helps a great deal to relieve vomiting. This method can also be tried for preventing the vomiting of food.

6. Those with nausea and vomiting should be instructed not to be nervous about their condition and to take proper rest.

Appended Formulas

1. *Shun Gan Yi Qi Tang (*from *Fu Qing Zhu Nu Ke [Fu Qing-zhu's Gynecology]):* Radix Panacis Ginseng (*Ren Shen*), Radix Angelicae Sinensis (*Dang Gui*), stir-fried Fructus Perillae Frutescentis (*Su Zi*),stir-fried Rhizoma Atractylodis Macrocephalae (*Bai Zhu*), Sclerotium Poriae Cocos (*Fu Ling*), wine stir-fried Radix Albus Paeoniae Lactiflorae (*Bai Shao*), Tuber Ophiopogonis Japonicae (*Mai Dong*), Fructus Amomi (*Sha Ren*), Massa Medica Fermentata (*Shen Qu*), Pericarpium Citri Reticulatae (*Chen Pi*), processed Rhizoma Pinelliae Ternatae (*Ban Xia*)

2. *Ren Shen Ju Pi Tang (*from *Zheng Zhi Zhun Sheng [Patterns & Treatments Norms & Criteria]):* Radix Panacis Ginseng (*Ren Shen*), Exocarpium Citri Grandis (*Ju Pi*), Sclerotium Rubrum Poriae Cocos (*Chi Ling*), stir-fried Rhizoma Atractylodis Macrocephalae (*Bai Zhu*), Tuber Ophiopogonis Japonicae (*Mai Dong*), Cortex Magnoliae Officinalis (*Hou Po*), Caulis In Taeniis Bambusae (*Zhu Ru*), Fructus Amomi (*Sha Ren*), Radix Glycyrrhizae (*Gan Cao*)

119

3. *Jia Wei Wen Dan Tang* (from *Yi Zong Jin Jian [Golden Mirror of Ancestral Medicine]*): Pericarpium Citri Reticulatae (*Chen Pi*), Rhizoma Pinelliae Ternatae (*Ban Xia*), Sclerotium Poriae Cocos (*Fu Ling*), Radix Glycyrrhizae (*Gan Cao*), Fructus Immaturus Citri Seu Ponciri (*Zhi Shi*), Caulis In Taeniis Bambusae (*Zhu Ru*), Radix Scutellariae Baicalensis (*Huang Qin*), Rhizoma Coptidis Chinensis (*Huang Lian*), Rhizoma Phragmitis Communis (*Lu Gen*), Tuber Ophiopogonis Japonicae (*Mai Dong*), uncooked Rhizoma Zingiberis (*Sheng Jiang*)

4. *Zhi Bai Di Huang Wan* (from *Yi Zong Jin Jian [Golden Mirror of Ancestral Medicine]*): prepared Radix Rehmanniae (*Shu Di*), Fructus Corni Officinalis (*Shan Zhu Yu*), Radix Dioscoreae Oppositae (*Shan Yao*), Sclerotium Poriae Cocos (*Fu Ling*), Cortex Radicis Moutan (*Dan Pi*), Rhizoma Alismatis (*Ze Xie*), Rhizoma Anemarrhenae (*Zhi Mu*), Cortex Phellodendri (*Huang Bai*)

5. *Zi Yin Jiang Ni Tang:* uncooked Concha Ostreae (*Mu Li*), uncooked Radix Albus Paeoniae Lactiflorae (*Bai Shao*), uncooked Radix Rehmanniae (*Sheng Di*), Fructus Lycii Chinensis (*Gou Qi Zi*), Fructus Corni Officinalis (*Shan Zhu Yu*), Radix Codonopsis Pilosulae (*Dang Shen*), Haemititum (*Dai Zhe Shi*), Radix Trichosanthis Kirlowii (*Tian Hua Fen*), Radix Angelicae Sinensis (*Dang Gui*), Plastrum Testudinis (*Gui Ban*), Lignum Aquilariae Agallochae (*Chen Xiang*)

6. *Zhu Ru Tang* (from *Da Sheng Yao Zhi [Essentials of Great Life]*): Ginger(-processed) Rhizoma Pinelliae Ternatae (*Ban Xia*), Caulis Perillae Frutescentis (*Su Gen*), Herba Agastachis Seu Pogostemi (*Huo Xiang*), Pericarpium Citri Reticulatae (*Chen Pi*), Radix Scutellariae Baicalensis (*Huang Qin*), Fructus Citri Seu Ponciri (*Zhi Ke*), stir-fried Radix Albus Paeoniae Lactiflorae (*Bai Shao*), Sclerotium Poriae Cocos (*Fu Ling*), Caulis In Taeniis Bambusae (*Zhu Ru*)

7. *Xiang Sha Liu Jun Zi Tang:* See Section Two, Chapter Four.

8. *Er Chen Tang* (from *Tai Ping Hui Min He Ji Ju Fang [Tai Ping Imperial Grace Formulary]*): Pericarpium Citri Reticulatae (*Chen Pi*), Rhizoma

Pinelliae Ternatae (*Ban Xia*), Sclerotium Poriae Cocos (*Fu Ling*), Radix Glycyrrhizae (*Gan Cao*)

Section Two

Abdominal Pain During Pregnancy (*Ren Shen Fu Tong*)

After becoming pregnant, if a woman experiences pain in her abdomen, this is called abdominal pain during pregnancy. The *Jin Gui Yao Lue (Essentials from the Golden Cabinet)* calls this *bao zu*, wrapper obstruction. This is because it results from obstruction and stagnation of the *bao mai*. This pain may be felt anywhere between the chest and abdomen, within the lower abdomen, or in the low back and abdominal areas.

Disease Causes, Disease Mechanisms

The *Jin Gui Yao Lue (Essentials from the Golden Cabinet)* says:

> In women who have been pregnant 6-7 months, there is a wiry pulse and fever. The fetus is well and grows. However, there is lower abdominal pain and aversion to cold, and the lower abdomen feels as if fanned. If it is extreme, the fetal viscus opens. *Fu Zi Tang* (Aconite Decoction) works for this viscus."

Another quotation says:

> Women may have leakage below. They may have half birth (*i.e.*, miscarriage) which causes continuous bleeding below which does not stop. If a pregnant woman precipitates blood, she may also have pain inside her abdomen. This is wrapper obstruction. *Jiao Ai Tang* (Donkey Skin Glue & Mugwort Decoction) rules this.

> Women who are pregnant may have pain within their abdomen. *Dang Gui Shao Yao San* (Dang Gui & Peony Powder) rules this.

121

This shows that the diseases causes, patterns, and treatment formulas and methods for abdominal pain during pregnancy are not all the same. In addition to qi and blood vacuity weakness and fetal viscus vacuity cold discussed above, in clinical practice, abdominal pain during pregnancy may be due wind cold food stagnation, depression and binding of the qi mechanism, and detriment and damage due to fall or strike.

Disease Patterns

Vacuity Cold

During pregnancy there is lower abdominal chilly pain, bodily cold, chilled limbs, possible superficial edema of the face and eyes, loose stools, a white, slimy or thin, white tongue coating, and a deep, weak pulse.

Qi Vacuity

There is low back and abdominal aching and pain accompanied by downward sagging and discomfort, essence spirit fatigue, a somber white facial complexion, shortness of breath, diminished appetite, dizziness, vertigo, a thin, white tongue coating with a pale or fat tongue, and a fine, weak or vacuous, large pulse.

Wind Cold Food Stagnation

There is epigastric and abdominal fullness and pain, much belching and burping, and diminished food and drink. In food stagnation, there is commonly acid eructation, chest and epigastric satiation and oppression, constipation or loose stools with a foul odor. Wind cold is commonly accompanied by aching and pain of the joints of the bones, head distention, headache, possible cough, possible fever, etc. The tongue coating is thin and white or white and slimy.

Qi Depression

There is lower abdominal distention and pain, tension, and discomfort, or chest and lateral costal pain, and essence spirit depression. If there is simultaneous depressive fire, there will be a tidal red facial complexion, headache, easy anger, a bitter taste in the mouth, a dry throat, dry stools, yellowish red urination, and fetal stirring restlessness. The tongue coating is thin and slimy or thin and yellow. The pulse is wiry.

Detriment & Damage by Fall or Strike

There is abdominal pain is caused by external injury radiating to the low back and abdomen. There is also fetal stirring restlessness or fetal stirring is diminished and weak. If severe, fetal stirring disappears.

Treatment

Vacuity Cold

One should warm the channels, nourish the blood, and quiet the fetus. The formula to use is *Jiao Ai Tang* (Donkey Skin Glue & Mugwort Decoction). If there is lower abdomen aversion to cold and the lower abdomen feels as if it were being fanned, one can use *Fu Zi Tang* (Aconite Decoction). If there is superficial edema of the face and eyes due to water dampness, the formula to use is *Dang Gui Shao Yao San* (Dang Gui & Peony Powder).

Qi Vacuity

One should boost the qi and supplementing vacuity, stop pain and quiet the fetus. The formula to use is *Bu Zhong Yi Qi Tang* (Supplement the Center & Boost the Qi Decoction).

Wind Cold Food Stagnation

For wind cold, one should resolve the exterior. The formula to use is *Zi Su Yin* (Perilla Drink) or *Jin Fei Cao San* (Herba Inulae Britannicae Powder).

123

For food stagnation, one should use *Ping Wei San* (Level the Stomach Powder).

Qi Depression

One should resolve depression and rectify the qi. The formula to use is *Suo Sha Yin* (Amomum Drink). If there is simultaneous depressive fire, one can use *Dan Zhi Xiao Yao San* (Moutan & Gardenia Rambling Powder).

Detriment & Damage due to Fall or Strike

One should supplement the qi and blood and quiet the fetal origin. If the pregnant woman's body is inclined toward blood vacuity, use *Jiao Ai Tang* (Donkey Skin Glue & Mugwort Decoction). If it is inclined toward qi vacuity, use *Bu Zhong Yi Qi Tang* (Supplement the Center & Boost the Qi Decoction). If qi and blood are both vacuous, use *Ba Zhen Tang* (Eight Pearls Decoction). To these can be added Cortex Eucommiae Ulmoidis (*Du Zhong*), Ramus Loranthi Seu Visci (*Sang Ji Sheng*), Radix Dipsaci (*Xu Duan*), Rhizoma Cibotii (*Gou Ji*), and Radix Albus Paeoniae Lactiflorae (*Bai Shao*) in order to secure the kidneys and quiet the fetus. If there is stasis, one can add ingredients which move stasis and stop pain, such as Resina Olibani (*Ru Xiang*), Resina Myrrhae (*Mo Yao*), and Lignum Sappan (*Su Mu*).

Explanation

1. If abdominal pain is due to detriment and damage by fall or strike during the early stages of pregnancy, one should take care that there is no sagging downward sensation in the lower abdomen and leakage of red (*i.e.*, blood). If this occurs after the fifth or sixth months of pregnancy, fetal movement should be closely monitored. Mild, weak fetal stirring or no stirring signifies that the fetus is not yet dead. One should add to the above formulas moving the qi medicinals such as Folium Artemisiae Argyii (*Ai Ye*), Rhizoma Cyperi Rotundi (*Xiang Fu*), and Fructus Amomi (*Sha Ren*) in order to regulate the qi and quiet the fetus. However, if the mother's tongue is blue, her abdomen is chilled, she has bad breath, and her pulse is

choppy, the decoction *Fu Shou San* (Buddha's Hand Powder) or other such abortive measures should be administered whenever suspected fetal death is confirmed by urine analysis or pelvic examination.

2. Abdominal pain during pregnancy requires immediate treatment. Otherwise, this may easily lead to the arising of fetal restlessness and, if severe, leakage and precipitation of blood, miscarriage, or fetal death within the abdomen.

Appended Formulas

1. *Jiao Ai Tang:* See Section Four, Chapter Four.

2. *Fu Zi Tang (*from *Shang Han Lun [Treatise on Damage Due to Cold]):* Radix Lateralis Praeparatus Aconiti Carmichaeli *(Fu Zi)*, Radix Panacis Ginseng *(Ren Shen)*, Rhizoma Atractylodis Macrocephalae *(Bai Zhu)*, Sclerotium Poriae Cocos *(Fu Ling)*, Radix Albus Paeoniae Lactiflorae *(Bai Shao)*

3. *Dang Gui Shao Yao San (*from *Jin Gui Yao Lue [Essentials from the Golden Cabinet]):* Radix Angelicae Sinensis *(Dang Gui)*, Radix Albus Paeoniae Lactiflorae *(Bai Shao)*, Radix Ligustici Wallichii *(Chuan Xiong)*, Sclerotium Poriae Cocos *(Fu Ling)*, Rhizoma Atractylodis Macrocephalae *(Bai Zhu)*, Rhizoma Alismatis *(Ze Xie)*

4. *Bu Zhong Yi Qi Tang:* See Section One, Chapter Four.

5. *Zi Su Yin:* Folium Perillae Frutescentis *(Su Ye)*, Pericarpium Arecae Catechu *(Da Fu Pi)*, Radix Albus Paeoniae Lactiflorae *(Bai Shao)*, Radix Codonopsis Pilosulae *(Dang Shen)*, Pericarpium Citri Reticulatae *(Chen Pi)*, Radix Angelicae Sinensis *(Dang Gui)*, Radix Glycyrrhizae *(Gan Cao)*, Bulbus Allii Fistulosi *(Cong Bai)*, uncooked Rhizoma Zingiberis *(Sheng Jiang)*

6. *Jin Fei Cao San (*from *Fu Ren Da Quan Liang Fang [A Great, Complete {Collection of} Fine Formulas for Women]):* Herba Inulae Britannicae *(Jin*

125

Fei Cao), Radix Peucedani (*Qian Hu*), Herba Seu Flos Schizonepetae Tenuifoliae (*Jing Jie*), Rhizoma Pinelliae Ternatae (*Ban Xia*), Herba Cum Radice Asari Seiboldi (*Xi Xin*), Sclerotium Poriae Cocos (*Fu Ling*), Radix Glycyrrhizae (*Gan Cao*)

7. *Ping Wei San (*from *Yi Zong Jin Jian [Golden Mirror of Ancestral Medicine]):* Rhizoma Atractylodis (*Cang Zhu*), Cortex Magnoliae Officinalis (*Hou Po*), Pericarpium Citri Reticulatae (*Chen Pi*), Fructus Amomi Tsaoko (*Cao Guo*), Fructus Citri Seu Ponciri (*Zhi Ke*), Massa Medica Fermentata (*Shen Qu*), Radix Glycyrrhizae (*Gan Cao*)

8. *Suo Sha Yin (*from *Nu Ke Zhi [Gynecology {As Clear As} the Fingers {in One's} Palm]):* 1.2g of powdered Fructus Amomi (*Sha Ren*) taken with water

9. *Dan Zhi Xiao Yao San (*from *Nu Ke Cuo Yao [Gathered Essentials of Gynecology]):* Radix Angelicae Sinensis (*Dang Gui*), Radix Albus Paeoniae Lactiflorae (*Bai Shao*), Radix Bupleuri (*Chai Hu*), Sclerotium Poriae Cocos (*Fu Ling*), Radix Glycyrrhizae (*Gan Cao*), Herba Menthae Haplocalycis (*Bo He*), Cortex Radicis Moutan (*Dan Pi*), Fructus Gardeniae Jasminoidis (*Shan Zhi*), Rhizoma Atractylodis Macrocephalae (*Bai Zhu*), baked Rhizoma Zingiberis (*Wei Jiang*)

10. *Ba Zhen Tang (*from *Zheng Zhi Zhun Sheng [Patterns & Treatments Norms & Criteria]):* See Section Four, Chapter Four.

Section Three

Fetal Stirring Restlessness (*Tai Dong Bu An*)

Fetal stirring restlessness mostly manifests itself clinically as low back soreness and abdominal pain. There may be lower abdominal downward sagging or possible red flow from the vaginal tract. These are not normal and diagnosis should be sought. Because individuals' bodies are not the same, the causes leading to the arising of this condition and their treatment

126

are also not the same. Therefore, interrogation or questioning is a necessary means for ascertaining the pattern and its cause and thus for giving treatment based on pattern discrimination. As soon as fetal stirring restlessness is noticed, the patient should be treated without delay so as to prevent miscarriage.

Disease Causes, Disease Mechanisms

After a woman become pregnant, if her qi and blood are full and sufficient and her body is strong and replete, yin and yang will be regulated and harmonious and this will lead to the fetal qi being quiet and secure. If qi and blood are not regulated or have suffered detriment and damage, this leads to fetal stirring restlessness, to the fetal qi counterflowing upward, to aching and pain within the abdomen, or to lower abdominal heaviness and sagging. If severe, there may be leakage of red. If these are not treated in time, there may be falling fetus and small birth or miscarriage. Chen Liang-fu says:

> During pregnancy there is fetal stirring restless. This is due to *chong* and *ren mai* vacuity, in which case the fetus is not replete.

The *chong* governs the sea of blood. The *ren* rules the uterus and fetus. If bedroom taxation damages the kidneys, if the mother's body is kidney qi vacuous, if spleen qi is vacuous and weak, or if there is detriment and damage due to fall or strike, the *chong* and *ren mai* may become vacuous and the fetal qi is not secure.

Disease Patterns

Kidney Vacuity

There is low back and knee soreness and stiffness, fetal stirring restlessness, fatigue and weakness of the body and limbs, dizziness, tinnitus, abdominal pain, possible downward sagging in the lower abdomen and leakage of red. The tongue is pale with a thin, white coating, and the pulse is deep, fine, and slippery.

127

Liver Depression

There is fetal stirring restlessness or red flowing from the vaginal tract, essence spirit depression, lateral costal distention and pain, belching and burping, diminished appetite, possible vomiting of bitter or sour, a thin, slimy tongue coating, and a wiry, slippery pulse.

Spleen Vacuity

There is fetal stirring during pregnancy and downward sagging, low back soreness, abdominal distention, loose stools, possible vomiting or diarrhea and, if severe, abdominal pain, a pale, fat tongue with a thin, slimy or thin, white coating, and a fine, slippery pulse.

Detriment & Damage Due to Fall or Strike

Due to loss of footing fall or strike, fall from a high place, or taxation damage beyond limit damaging the fetal origin, there is pain within the abdomen. If severe, blood is precipitated and does not stop. Outwardly one looks as if they are about to fall.

Strike by Toxins (*i.e.*, Poisoning)

The pregnant woman has eaten toxic foodstuffs. If mild, there is damage and stirring of the fetal qi and fetal stirring restlessness. If severe, there is lockjaw, epilepsy, inability of the mouth to speak, rigidity of both upper extremities, spontaneous sweating, slight fever, and various other symptoms of poisoning. The pulse is floating and soft. Some of these symptoms are quite similar to wind stroke during pregnancy.

Vacuity Cold

There is fetal stirring restlessness with edema, vomiting, nausea, a desire for heat and fear of cold, possible chilly pain in the epigastrium or abdomen. The pulse is deep and fine.

Heat Pattern

Three is fetal stirring restlessness, occasional abdominal pain, a subjective sensation of vexatious heat, red lips, red tongue, possible thirst or dry mouth, red urine, and a slippery, rapid pulse.

Treatment

Kidney Vacuity

One should supplement the kidneys and quiet the fetus. The formula to use is mainly *Di Huang Tang* (Rehmannia Decoction) or *An Dian Er Tian Tang* (Quiet & Settle the Two Heavens Decoction). If signs of leakage of red appear, to prevent falling fetus, one can use *An Tai San* (Quiet the Fetus Powder) or *Xiong Gui Jiao Ai Tang* (Ligusticum & Dang Gui Donkey Skin Glue & Mugwort Decoction).

Liver Depression

One should course the liver, resolve depression, and quiet the fetus. the formula to use is *Xiao Yao San* (Rambling Powder) or *Jie Yu Tang* (Resolve Depression Decoction).

Spleen Vacuity

One should fortify the spleen, boost the qi, and quiet the fetus. The formula to use is *Yuan Tu Gu Tai Tang* (Aid Earth & Secure the Fetus Decoction) or *Xiang Sha Liu Jun Zi Tang* (Saussurea & Amomum Six Gentlemen Decoction).

Detriment & Damage Due to Fall or Strike

Such patients must be coped with flexibly on a case to case basis. It is common to find that those in whom the fetus origin is tight and secure will not manifest any specific abnormalities even if a fall or strike does occur to them. While in those with protracted of qi and blood deficiency, the fetus may stir due to even a minor fall or strike. In such cases, it is preferable to greatly supplement the qi and blood but avoiding those ingredients which move stasis. The formula that is mainly for this is *Juo Sun An Tai Tang* (Stem Detriment & Quiet the Fetus Decoction). If there is excessive bleeding, one can use *E Jiao San* (Donkey Skin Glue Powder) to stop bleeding and quiet the fetus or *Xiong Gui Tang* (Ligusticum & Dang Gui Decoction) to regulate and treat. This will lead to fetal stirring becoming quiet. However, the tongue and pulse signs associated with fetal stirring should be closely monitored so that immediate measures can be taken in time in order to forestall fetal death and in order to protect the mother's quiet.

Food Poisoning

The formula to use is *San Wu Jie Du Tang* (Three Materials Resolve Toxins Decoction) or *Bai Bian Dou San* (Dolichos Powder) to resolve toxins and quiet the fetus. If the fetus has already died, one can administer *Duo Ming Wan* (Seize the Destiny Pills) to precipitate the fetus.

Extremes of Cold or Heat

For extreme cold, the formula to use is *Bai Zhu San* (Atractylodes Powder). For heat patterns, use *Dang Gui San* (Dang Gui Powder) to nourish the blood and clear heat.

The treatment of this disease depends upon its cause. If the mother is diseased and the fetus stirs, treat the mother's disease and the fetus will automatically be quieted. If the fetus is not secure and therefore the mother is diseased, quiet the fetus and the mother will automatically be quieted.

Explanation

1. For fetal stirring restlessness and appearance of leakage of red, typically one can mainly use the two formulas *An Tai San* (Quiet the Fetus Powder)

and *Jiao Ai Tang* (Donkey Skin Glue & Mugwort Decoction). If the precipitated blood is excessive, one can add Radix Panacis Ginseng (*Ren Shen*). If there is qi vacuity heaviness and sagging, one can use *Bu Zhong Yi Qi Tang* (Supplement the Center & Boost the Qi). These can be added to or subtracted from following the pattern.

2. Based on our predecessors' statements that quieting the fetus mostly depends on the spleen and stomach, one can commonly administer formulas for fortifying the spleen and clearing heat and the fetus will automatically be quieted. Dan-xi has said that Radix Scutellariae Baicalensis (*Huang Qin*) and Rhizoma Atractylodis Macrocephalae (*Bai Zhu*) are sage-like medicinals for quieting the fetus. However, they should be carefully considered following the person's body, the cause, and the progression of the disease. Radix Scutellariae Baicalensis (*Huang Qin*) is used for internal heat patterns. If there is qi vacuity and internal cold and it is used, it can cause an adverse effect on the patient. Rhizoma Atractylodis Macrocephalae (*Bai Zhu*) is good for supplementing the spleen and quieting the fetus. However, its nature is drying and closes the qi. If there is yin vacuity or qi stagnation in a person, its use should be carefully considered. In a word, because in pregnant women, cold and heat, vacuity and repletion are not all the same, medicinals should follow the pattern presented.

Appended Formulas

1. *Di Huang Tang (*from *Xiao Er Yao Zheng Zhi Jue [Frank Tricks of the Trade {in the Use of} Pediatric Medicinals & Patterns]):* Prepared Radix Rehmanniae (*Shu Di*), Fructus Corni Officinalis (*Shan Zhu Yu*), Radix Dioscoreae Oppositae (*Shan Yao*), Cortex Radicis Moutan (*Dan Pi*), Sclerotium Poriae Cocos (*Fu Ling*), Rhizoma Alismatis (*Ze Xie*)

2. *An Dian Er Tian Tang (*from *Fu Qing Zhu Nu Ke (Fu Qing-zhu's Gynecology]):* Radix Panacis Ginseng (*Ren Shen*), prepared Radix Rehmanniae (*Shu Di*), Rhizoma Atractylodis Macrocephalae (*Bai Zhu*), Radix

131

Dioscoreae Oppositae (*Shan Yao*), Fructus Corni Officinalis (*Shan Zhu Yu*), Cortex Eucommiae Ulmoidis (*Du Zhong*), Fructus Lycii Chinensis (*Gou Qi Zi*), Semen Dolichoris Lablab (*Bian Dou*), mix-fried Radix Glycyrrhizae (*Gan Cao*)

3. *An Tai San (*from *Bu Yi Fang [Supplementing Lost Formulas]):* Prepared Radix Rehmanniae (*Shu Di*), Folium Artemisiae Argyii (*Ai Ye*), Radix Albus Paeoniae Lactiflorae (*Bai Shao*), Radix Ligustici Wallichii (*Chuan Xiong*), Radix Astragali Membranacei (*Huang Qi*), Gelatinum Corii Asini (*E Jiao*), Radix Angelicae Sinensis (*Dang Gui*), Radix Glycyrrhizae (*Gan Cao*), Radix Sanguisorbae (*Di Yu*), Sclerotium Poriae Cocos (*Fu Ling*). Add Rhizoma Zingiberis (*Jiang*) and Fructus Zizyphi Jujubae (*Zao*) and decoct in water. Or add Cortex Eucommiae Ulmoidis (*Du Zhong*) and Radix Dipsaci (*Chuan Duan*).

4. *Xiong Gui Jiao Ai Tang (*from *Jin Gui Yao Lue [Essentials from the Golden Cabinet]):* Uncooked Radix Rehmanniae (*Sheng Di*), Radix Angelicae Sinensis (*Dang Gui*), Radix Ligustici Wallichii (*Chuan Xiong*), Radix Albus Paeoniae Lactiflorae (*Bai Shao*), Gelatinum Corii Asini (*E jiao*), Folium Artemisiae Argyii (*Ai Ye*)

5. *Xiao Yao San:* See Section Two, Chapter Four.

6. *Jie Yu Tang (*from *Fu Qing Zhu Nu Ke [Fu Qing-zhu's Gynecology]):* Radix Panacis Ginseng (*Ren Shen*), Rhizoma Atractylodis Macrocephalae (*Bai Zhu*), Sclerotium Poriae Cocos (*Fu Ling*), Radix Angelicae Sinensis (*Dang Gui*), Radix Albus Paeoniae Lactiflorae (*Bai Shao*), Fructus Citri Seu Ponciri (*Zhi Ke*), Fructus Amomi (*Sha Ren*), Fructus Gardeniae Jasminoidis (*Shan Zhi*), Herba Menthae Haplocalycis (*Bo He*)

7. *Yuan Tu Gu Tai Tang (*from *Fu Qing Zhu Nu Ke [Fu Qing-zhu's Gynecology]):* Radix Panacis Ginseng (*Ren Shen*), Rhizoma Atractylodis Macrocephalae (*Bai Zhu*), Radix Dioscoreae Oppositae (*Shan Yao*), Cortex Cinnamomi (*Rou Gui*), Radix Lateralis Praeparatus Aconiti Carmichaeli (*Fu Zi*), Radix Dipsaci (*Xu Duan*), Cortex Eucommiae Ulmoidis (*Du Zhong*), Fructus Corni Officinalis (*Shan Zhu Yu*), Fructus Lycii Chinensis

(*Gou Qi Zi*), Semen Cuscutae (*Tu Si Zi*), Fructus Amomi (*Sha Ren*), Radix Glycyrrhizae (*Gan Cao*)

8. *Xiang Sha Liu Jun Zi Tang:* See Section Two, Chapter Four.

9. *Juo Sun An Tai Tang* (from *Fu Qing Zhu Nu Ke [Fu Qing-zhu's Gynecology]):* Radix Angelicae Sinensis (*Dang Gui*), Radix Albus Paeoniae Lactiflorae (*Bai Shao*), uncooked Radix Rehmanniae (*Sheng Di*), Rhizoma Atractylodis Macrocephalae (*Bai Zhu*), mix-fried Radix Glycyrrhizae (*Zhi Gan Cao*), Radix Panacis Ginseng (*Ren Shen*), Lignum Sappan (*Su Mu*), Resina Olibani (*Ru Xiang*), Resina Myrrhae (*Mo Yao*)

10. *E Jiao San* (from *Zheng Zhi Zhun Sheng [Patterns & Treatments Norms & Criteria]):* Prepared Radix Rehmanniae (*Shu Di*), Radix Albus Paeoniae Lactiflorae (*Bai Shao*), Folium Artemisiae Argyii (*Ai Ye*), Radix Angelicae Sinensis (*Dang Gui*), mix-fried Radix Astragali Membranacei (*Huang Qi*), Radix Glycyrrhizae (*Gan Cao*), stir-fried Gelatinum Corii Asini (*E Jiao*), uncooked Rhizoma Zingiberis (*Sheng Jiang*), Fructus Zizyphi Jujubae (*Da Zao*)

11. *Xiong Gui Tang* (from *Yi Lei Yuan Cheng [The Origin of the Creation of the Ramparts of Medicine]):* Radix Ligustici Wallichii (*Chuan Xiong*), Radix Angelicae Sinensis (*Dang Gui*)

12. *San Wu Jie Du Tang:* Uncooked Radix Glycyrrhizae (*Gan Cao*), Semen Glycinis Hispidae (*Hei Dou*), Folium Lophatheri Gracilis (*Dan Zhu Ye*). Use equal parts of these medicinals, decoct in water, and administer.

13. *Bai Bian Dou San* (from *Shen Shi Zun Sheng Shu [Master Shen's Writings on Respecting Life]):* Grind 100g of peeled Semen Dolichoris Lablab (*Bian Dou*) into powder and take after mixing with water.

14. *Duo Ming Wan* (from *Ji Yin Gang Mu [Detailed Outline of Yin]):* Cortex Radicis Moutan (*Dan Pi*), Semen Pruni Persicae (*Tao Ren*), Sclerotium Poriae Cocos (*Fu Ling*), Radix Albus Paeoniae Lactiflorae (*Bai Shao*), Cortex Cinnamomi (*Gui Xin*)

133

15. *Bai Zhu San (*from *Jin Gui Yao Lue [Essentials from the Golden Cabinet]):* Rhizoma Atractylodis Macrocephalae (*Bai Zhu*), Radix Ligustici Wallichii (*Chuan Xiong*), Fructus Zanthoxyli Bungeani (*Chuan Jiao*), Concha Ostreae (*Mu Li*)

16. *Dang Gui San (*from *Jin Gui Yao Lue (Essentials from the Golden Cabinet]):* Radix Angelicae Sinensis (*Dang Gui*), Radix Albus Paeoniae Lactiflorae (*Bai Shao*), Rhizoma Atractylodis Macrocephalae (*Bai Zhu*), Radix Scutellariae Baicalensis (*Huang Qin*), Radix Ligustici Wallichii (-*Chuan Xiong*)

Section Four

Vaginal Leakage Precipitating Blood (*Tai Lou Xia Xue*)

Vaginal leakage precipitating blood refers to not very great fetal stirring during pregnancy, no low back soreness or abdominal pain, but blood flowing from the vaginal tract. Some women may also still have regular periods despite conception. This is called stimulated menstruation or exuberant fetus. Typically, after 4-5 months, following the growth of the fetal child, it needs an increasing amount of construction and nourishment to sustain and develop it. Therefore, the menstrual movement also ceases and stops. Generally, this does not cause detriment to the fetal child.

Disease Causes, Disease Mechanisms

This disease is mostly seen due to blood heat, wind heat, and spleen vacuity. It may also be due to qi and blood transportation and movement not abiding in its normal pathways. In addition, it may be due to blood vacuity not being able to supply the fetus and thus the blood precipitates downward.

Disease Patterns

Blood Heat

There is leakage and precipitation of blood which is colored deep red or is excessive in volume. It may look like red bean juice. There may also be low back and abdominal soreness and pain, heart vexation, and easy anger. The tongue coating is thin and white or yellow and slimy, and the pulse is wiry and rapid.

Wind Heat

There is fetal leakage and precipitated blood. The body is cold but there is generalized fever. There is head distention and dizziness, the mouth is dry, and there is a bitter flavor. The urination is yellowish red. The tongue coating is thin and white or thin and yellow. The pulse is floating and rapid.

Spleen/Stomach Vacuity Weakness

There is essence spirit fatigue, bodily emaciation and weakness, devitalized appetite, chest and diaphragmatic inhibition, non-replete stools or defecating numerous times, fetal leakage and precipitated blood like bean juice or possibly like glue, a sallow yellow facial complexion, a pale, fat tongue with a thin, white coating, and a weak pulse.

Blood Vacuity

There is fetal leakage and precipitated blood that is fresh red in color or pale, dizziness, heart palpitations, evening sleep not deep, possible bodily cold, or heat and dry throat. The tongue coating is thin and white, the tongue is pale, and the pulse is fine and rapid.

Concretion Disease

The pregnant woman has concretion disease (*i.e.*, abdominal mass). After being pregnant for not quite 3 whole months, there is leakage and precipi-

135

tation which does not stop. This is accompanied by lower abdominal tension, low back soreness, lack of moisture in the skin, a lusterless facial complexion, a thin, white tongue coating with possible static spots, and a fine, choppy pulse.

Treatment

Blood Heat

One should clear heat and cool the blood, stop bleeding and quiet the fetus. The formula to use is *E Jiao Tang* (Donkey Skin Glue Decoction) or *Jia Wei Xiao Yao San* (Added Flavors Rambling Powder).

Wind Heat

One should course wind and clear heat, stop bleeding and quiet the fetus. The formula to use is *Fang Feng Huang Qin Tang* (Ledebouriella & Scutellaria Decoction) or *Yu Feng San* (Cure Wind Powder).

Spleen/Stomach Vacuity Weakness

One should supplement and boost the spleen and stomach. The formula to use is *Bu Zhong Yi Qi Tang* (Supplement the Center & Boost the Qi Decoction) or *Zu Qi Bu Lou Tang* (Assist the Qi & Supplement Leakage Decoction).

Blood Vacuity

One should nourish the blood, stop bleeding, and quiet the fetus. The formula to use is *Er Huang San* (Two Yellows Decoction). If there is leakage and precipitation with abdominal pain, *Jiao Ai Tang* (Donkey Skin Glue & Mugwort Decoction) rules this.

Concretion Disease

One should dispel stasis, disperse concretion, and stop bleeding. The formula to use is *Gui Zhi Fu Ling Wan* (Cinnamon Twig & Poria Pills).

Explanation

1. Fetal leakage should be distinguished from (both) stimulated menstruation and hematuria. Stimulated menstruation has already been discussed above. Hematuria refers to blood in the urine caused by urinary hot blood and the downward drive of pathogenic damp heat. The blood in this case is discharged from the urethra and therefore is always visible (in the urine).

2. Carbonized ingredients are always found as components of prescriptions for this condition. For example, carbonized Radix Rehmanniae and carbonized crown of Radix Angelicae Sinensis (*Dang Gui*) are used for cultivating the blood. Carbonized Cacumen Biotae and Radix Sanguisorbae are used for clearing heat.

3. Miscarriage most typically occurs because of the blood's inability to nourish and support the fetus after constant hemorrhage. As soon as retarded growth of the fetus is detected, scores of decoctions of *Ba Zhen Tang* plus Radix Panacis Ginseng (*Ren Shen*) and Radix Astragali Membranacei (*Huang Qi*) can revitalize the fetus.

4. For the sake of correct diagnosis, it is necessary to intensively inquire about the exact duration and volume of bleeding. The fetus is typically in jeopardy when the duration or volume of bleeding exceed that of past occurrences (*i.e.* increases noticeably). Examination of the fetus can be made by means of urine analysis during the early stages of pregnancy or by comparison of the parameters of fetal movement, heart tones, and abdominal girth of the expectant mother from the time of conception. In short, it is important to obtain evidence showing that the fetus is still alive before prescribing medicines for protecting the fetus and stopping leakage.

5. Pregnant women should be instructed not to climb heights, engage in sex, eat peppery foods, or take decoctions accelerating blood circulation. They should pay close attention to a well-regulated lifestyle.

Appended Formulas

1. *E Jiao Tang (*from *Yi Zong Jin Jian [Golden Mirror of Ancestral Medicine]):* Radix Angelicae Sinensis (*Dang Gui*), Radix Ligustici Wallichii (*Chuan Xiong*), Radix Albus Paeoniae Lactiflorae (*Bai Shao*), uncooked Radix Rehmanniae (*Sheng Di*), Gelatinum Corii Asini (*E Jiao*), Fructus Gardeniae Jasminoidis (*Shan Zhi*), Cacumen Biotae Orientalis (*Ce Bai Ye*), Radix Scutellariae Baicalensis (*Huang Qin*)

2. *Jia Wei Xiao Yao San:* See Section One, Chapter Four.

3. *Fang Feng Huang Qin Tang (*from *Fu Ren Da Quan Liang Fang [A Great, Complete {Collection of} Fine Formulas for Women]):* stir-fried, scorched Radix Scutellariae Baicalensis (*Huang Qin*), Radix Ledebouriellae Sesloidis (*Fang Feng*)

4. *Yu Feng San* (also know as *Yu Feng Tang;* from *Hua Yuan Hua Fang [Hua Yuan-hua's Formulas]):* Carbonized Herba Seu Flos Schizonepetae Tenuifoliae (*Jing Jie*), stir-fred Semen Glycinis Hispidae (*Hei Dou*), ground into powder and taken with wine.

5. *Bu Zhong Yi Qi Tang:* See Section Two, Chapter Four.

6. *Zu Qi Bu Lou Tang (*from *Fu Qing Zhu Nu Ke [Fu Qing-zhu's Gynecology]):* Radix Panacis Ginseng (*Ren Shen*), stir-fried Radix Albus Paeoniae Lactiflorae (*Bai Shao*, stir-fried Radix Scutellariae Baicalensis (*Huang Qin*), stir-fried, blackened uncooked Radix Rehmanniae (*Sheng Di*), Herba Leonuri Heterophylli (*Yi Mu Cao*), Radix Dipsaci (*Xu Duan*), Radix Glycyrrhizae (*Gan Cao*)

7. *Er Huang San (*from *Fu Ren Da Quan Liang Fang [A Great, Complete {Collection of} Fine Formulas for Women]):* Powdered Radix Rehmanniae

(*Sheng Di*), powdered prepared Radix Rehmanniae (*Shu di*), equal parts. Take 9g each time with a decoction of Rhizoma Atractylodis Macrocephalae (*Bai Zhu*) and Fructus Citri Seu Ponciri (*Zhi Ke*) before meals. Or take pills made of Radix Rehmanniae (*Sheng Di*) and prepared Radix Rehmanniae (*Shu Di*) instead.

8. *Jiao Ai Tang:* See Section Four, Chapter Four.

9. *Gui Zhi Fu Ling Wan (*from *Jin Gui Yao Lue [Essentials from the Golden Cabinet]):* Ramulus Cinnamomi (*Gui Zhi*), Sclerotium Poriae Cocos (*Fu Ling*), Cortex Radicis Moutan (*Dan Pi*), Semen Pruni Persicae (*Tao Ren*), Radix Rubrus Paeoniae Lactiflorae (*Chi Shao*)

Section Five

Falling Fetus & Small Birth (*Duo Tai Xiao Chan*)

If a pregnant woman gives birth before sufficient months, this is called falling fetus or small birth. Falling fetus and small birth differ form each other in several ways. If a woman gives birth after 5-7 months when the fetus has already formed, this is small birth. If this occurs within 3 months when the fetus is not formed, this is called falling fetus. In other words, if delivery occurs within 16 weeks of pregnancy, this is called flowing fetus (*i.e.*, miscarriage). If this occurs after 28 weeks, this is called small birth. If birth occurs after 7 months but before sufficient months (*i.e.*, full term), this is called early birth.

Disease Causes, Disease Mechanisms

This disease mostly results from fetal stirring restlessness and fetal leakage with precipitated blood. Thus its causes are mostly the same as fetal stirring restless and fetal leakage with precipitated blood. these have been described above. Clinically, it is often noticed that, after falling fetus and small birth, the lochia is either excessive or does not stop. Typically, if the

139

lochia is scanty, this is accompanied by abdominal pain. The former is mostly due to the *chong* and *ren mai* having suffered detriment and damage and not being able to contain the blood or static blood not permitting new blood to return to the channels. The latter is due to blood congelation not moving and vanquished blood closing and obstructing or external cold evils congealing.

Disease Patterns

Chong & *Ren* Detriment & Damage

After falling fetus or small birth, blood precipitates and does not stop but is like a flood. If severe, there is dizziness and fainting or dribbling and dripping for many days which does not stop. There is also low back soreness and slack limbs, a somber white facial complexion, abdominal pain which likes pressure, a pale tongue with a scanty coating, and a vacuous, weak pulse.

Static Blood Internally Obstructing

After falling fetus or small birth, there is precipitation of blood which does not stop or which dribbles and drips for many days. There is also abdominal pain which refuses pressure, slightly bluish gums, a thin, white tongue coating, a possibly purplish tongue, and a fine, choppy pulse image.

Blood Congelation Not Moving

After falling fetus or small birth, the lochia is scanty or does not descend. However, there is lower abdominal hardness and pain which refuses pressure. The pain's force is very severe. The tongue is a stagnant blue and the pulse is deep and choppy.

Treatment

Chong & *Ren* Detriment & Damage

One should greatly supplement the qi and blood. The formula to use is *Shi Sheng Tang* (Ten Sages Powder) or *Gui Pi Tang* (Restore the Spleen Decoction) plus carbonized Petiolus Trachycarpi (*Chen Zong Tan*), Crinis Carbonisatus (*Xue Yu Tan*), and carbonized Rhizoma Dryopteridis Crassirhizomae (*Guan Zhong*).

Static Blood Internally Obstructing

One should dispel stasis and engender the new. The formula to use is *Shi Xiao San* (Sudden Smile Powder) and *Sheng Hua Tang* (Engendering & Transforming Decoction) plus Radix Achyranthis Bidentatae (*Niu Xi*), Radix Albus Paeoniae Lactiflorae (*Bai Shao*), and Herba Leonuri Heterophylli (*Yi Mu Cao*). In addition, Radix Pseudoginseng (*San Qi*) is ground into fine powder and swallowed together with this decoction.

Blood Congelation Not Moving

If static blood obstructs internally, use the above same treatment methods. If there is external contraction of wind cold evils causing this, then, in order to mainly warm the channels and scatter cold, use the formula *Wen Jing Tang* (Warm the Menses Decoction).

Explanation

1. The condition of small birth is typically preceded by fetal stirring restlessness, leakage of red and spotting, abdominal tension and pain, and lower abdominal sagging with the subsequent appearance of more intense pain, lumbosacral soreness or severe abdominal distention. Blood flow becomes more copious and a sticky fluid is precipitated. however, there is not always severe abdominal pain. If stirring fetus is due to fall or strike

141

detriment and damage, first there is the appearance of low back soreness and abdominal pain and later there is flowing blood and the precipitated fetus.

2. Based on clinical experience, if before small birth occurs the pregnant woman experiences abdominal pain and flowing blood which may be copious but does not experience low back soreness or pain, medicinals can be used and treatment is effective. However, if there is low back soreness and severe pain, even though precipitated blood is not excessive and the abdomen does not have severe pain, treatment with medicinals is not able to get a good effect. Therefore, previous persons have said:

> Women's kidneys are attached to the uterus and the low back is the mansion of the kidneys. Low back pain leads to falling and cannot be prevented.

Thus pregnant women who experience low back soreness must receive early treatment. If there is low back soreness, this may easily lead to the arising of miscarriage.

3. After small birth, the body should be properly nourished. Otherwise this may easily lead to the arising of various debility weakness conditions, such as low back soreness, dizziness, lack of the strength in the limbs and body, soreness and pain of the sinews and bones, etc.

4. In order to prevent small birth, it is essential to pay attention to bedroom affairs and overwork or small birth may occur. This is why bedroom affairs and overtaxation are prohibited. Clinically this is commonly seen.

Appended Formulas

1. *Shi Sheng San:* Radix Panacis Ginseng (*Ren Shen*), Radix Astragali Membranacei (*Huang Qi*), Rhizoma Atractylodis Macrocephalae (*Bai Zhu*), prepared Radix Rehmanniae (*Shu Di*), Fructus Amomi (*Sha Ren*), carbonized Radix Angelicae Sinensis (*Dang Gui*), Radix Ligustici

Wallichii (*Chuan Xiong*), stir-fried Radix Albus Paeoniae Lactiflorae (*Bai Shao*), Radix Dipsaci (*Xu Duan*), Radix Glycyrrhizae (*Gan Cao*)

2. *Gui Pi Tang:* See Section One, Chapter Four.

3. *Shi Xiao San:* See Section Ten, Chapter Four.

4. *Sheng Hua Tang (*from *Fu Qing Zhu Nu Ke [Fu Qing-zhu's Gynecology]):* Whole Radix Angelicae Sinensis (*Quan Dang Gui*), Radix Ligustici Wallichii (*Chuan Xiong*), Semen Pruni Persicae (*Tao Ren*), blast-fried Rhizoma Zingiberis (*Pao Jiang*), mix-fried Radix Glycyrrhizae (*Zhi Gan Cao*)

5. *Wen Jing Tang:* See Section Six, Chapter Four.

Section Six

Slippery Fetus (*Hua Tai*) (*i.e.*, Habitual Miscarriage [*Man Xing Liu Chan*])

Repeated falling fetus or small birth more than 3 times either successively or *in toto* is called slippery fetus. In modern medicine, this is called habitual miscarriage. However, in clinical practice, treatment methods for ensuring an easy birth are also called *hua tai*. For instance, the *Fu Ren Da Quan Liang Fang (A Great, Complete [Collection of} Fine Formulas for Women)* has *Hua Tai Tang* (Slippery Fetus Decoction). Thus there are two meanings of this term.

Disease Causes, Disease Mechanisms

The cause of this disease is similar to that of falling fetus and small birth in that it is mainly due to a weak natural endowment, qi and blood deficiency detriment, undisciplined bedroom affairs, and detriment and damage due to fall or strike causing qi and blood vacuity and debility. Thus the qi and blood is not able to nourish or gather the fetus. The kidney does not secure and the spleen qi does not contain. Therefore there are repeated miscarriages. In addition, blood heat easily stirs the fetus. Hence blood heat and vacuity are not uncommonly seen in clinical practice.

Disease Patterns

Qi & Blood Vacuity Weakness

As soon as there is pregnancy, there is commonly falling fetus, there is falling fetus after several months, or there is delivery before sufficient months. After 1 time of falling fetus/small birth, every other time there is pregnancy there is automatically falling. This is accompanied by bodily fatigue, dizziness, and vertigo which are mostly due to qi and blood dual vacuity. If there are heart palpitations and insomnia, this commonly pertains to blood vacuity. If there is torpid intake, slack limbs, abdominal distention, and loose stools, this is mainly due to spleen vacuity. If commonly there is a felling of low back soreness, frequent, clear urination, and clear, watery *dai xia*, this is mainly due to kidney vacuity. The tongue is pale with a thin, white coating. The pulse image is mostly vacuous and weak. The *chi* or foot pulse is mostly seen as vacuous and weak.

Blood Heat & Vacuity

Each time the woman gets pregnant there is commonly miscarriage. The cheeks of the face are flushed red and there is oral thirst leading to drinking. The stools are dry and there is low back soreness which is due to kidney vacuity, blood heat. the *chi* or foot pulse is large and without force.

Treatment

Qi & Blood Vacuity Weakness

Treatment should be based on a discrimination of patterns in turn based on an analysis of the qi, blood, spleen, and kidneys.

Qi & Blood Dual Vacuity: One should supplement and boost the qi and blood. In order to control the pregnant woman's body, the formula to use is (Zhang) Jing-yue's *Tai Yuan Yin* (Fetal Origin Drink). If the fetal origin is not secure, use large amounts of Rhizoma Atractylodis Macrocephalae (*Bai Zhu*) and add Radix Dioscoreae Oppositae (*Shan Yao*) and *Wei Xi Wan* (Impressive Might Joy Pills). If there is severe qi aspect vacuity, then use double amounts of Rhizoma Atractylodis Macrocephalae (*Bai Zhu*) with Radix Astragali Membranacei (*Huang Qi*). If vacuity is mixed with cold, add blast-fried Rhizoma Zingiberis (*Pao Jiang*). If vacuity is mixed with heat, add Radix Scutellariae Baicalensis (*Huang Qin*). Or one may use *Tai Shan Pan Shi San* (Tai Shan Building Stone Powder) or *Shi Quan Da Bu Tang* (Ten [Ingredients] Completely & Greatly Supplementing Decoction).

Predominant Blood Vacuity: One should nourish the blood and quiet the fetus. The formula to use is *Jiao Ai Tang* (Donkey Skin Glue & Mugwort Decoction).

Predominant Spleen Vacuity: One should fortify the spleen and quiet the fetus. The formula to use is *Qian Jin Bao Tao Wan* (*Thousand [Pieces of] Gold* Protect the Fetus Pills).

Predominant Kidney Vacuity: One should supplement the kidneys and attach the fetus. The formula to use is *Du Zhong Wan* (Eucommia Pills) or *Liu Wei Di Huang Wan* (Six Flavors Rehmannia Pills) plus Cortex Eucommiae Ulmoidis (*Du Zhong*), Radix Dipsaci (*Xu Duan*), Gelatinum Corii Asini (*E Jiao*), and Fructus Schizandrae Chinensis (*Wu Wei Zi*) to regulate and treat.

Blood Heat & Vacuity

One should clear heat and supplement vacuity. The formula to use is *Dang Gui San* (Dang Gui Powder) or *Huang Qin Bai Zhu Tang* (Scutellaria & Atractylodes Decoction). If there is kidney vacuity and blood heat, one should use *Liang Tai Yin* (Cool the Fetus Drink). If replete heat is severe, add Cortex Phellodendri (*Huang Bai*).

Explanation

1. This disease requires preventive treatment. The patient is advised to use contraceptives since they should not become pregnant for 1 year after their last miscarriage. After becoming pregnant, she should seek medical advice before taking any medicinals in order to determine what regulating treatment is necessary for prevention. Even if not pregnant, she should also be treated before and after each menstruation with different medicinals to regulate and rectify.

2. In this disease is vitally important to distinguish between vacuity and repletion, hot and cold, so that medicinals match the pattern. If there are no hot or cold symptoms apparent, one can use *Tai Yuan Yin* (Fetal Origin Drink) plus Sclerotium Pararadicis Poriae Cocos (*Fu Shen*), Radix Dipsaci (*Xu Duan*), and Ramus Loranthi Seu Visci (*Sang Ji Sheng*). Take 3-5 *ji* each monthly regularly and the clinical results are typically effective.

3. The use of *Tai Shan Pan Shi San* (*Tai Shan* Building Stone Powder) with additions and subtractions is quite effective in the treatment of qi and blood dual vacuity habitual miscarriage. It is mentioned in the ancient medical literature.

4. Radix Angelicae Sinensis (*Dang Gui*) and Radix Ligustici Wallichii (*Chuan Xiong*) are yang within the blood medicinals and have leading the blood and stirring the blood properties. Therefore they should be handled with great care in those with slippery fetus.

Appended Formulas

1. *Tai Yuan Yin* (from *Jing Yue Quan Shu [Jing-yue's Complete Writings]*): Radix Panacis Ginseng (*Ren Shen*), Radix Angelicae Sinensis (*Dang Gui*), Cortex Eucommiae Ulmoidis (*Du Zhong*), Radix Albus Paeoniae Lactiflorae (*Bai Shao*), prepared Radix Rehmanniae (*Shu Di*), Rhizoma Atractylodis Macrocephalae (*Bai Zhu*), Pericarpium Citri Reticulatae (*Chen Pi*), Radix Glycyrrhizae (*Gan Cao*)

2. *Wei Xi Wan:* Sclerotium Poriae Cocos (*Fu Ling*), Yellow Wax (*Huang La*)

3. *Tai Shan Pan Shi Tang* (from *Jing Yue Quan Shu [Jing-yue's Complete Writings]*): Radix Panacis Ginseng (*Ren Shen*), Radix Astragali Membranacei (*Huang Qi*), Radix Angelicae Sinensis (*Dang Gui*), Radix Dipsaci (*Xu Duan*), Radix Scutellariae Baicalensis (*Huang Qin*), Radix Ligustici Wallichii (*Chuan Xiong*), Radix Albus Paeoniae Lactiflorae (*Bai Shao*), prepared Radix Rehmanniae (*Shu Di*), Rhizoma Atractylodis Macrocephalae (*Bai Zhu*), mix-fried Radix Glycyrrhizae (*Zhi Gan Cao*), Fructus Oryzae Glutinosae (*Nuo Mi*)

4. *Shi Quan Da Bu Tang:* See Section Five, Chapter Four.

5. *Jiao Ai Tang:* See Section Four, Chapter Four

6. *Qian Jin Bao Tai Wan* (from *Qian Jin Fang [Formulas {Worth a} Thousand {Pieces of} Gold]*): Earth stir-fried Rhizoma Atractylodis Macrocephalae (*Bai Zhu*), ginger juice stir-fried prepared Radix Rehmanniae (*Shu Di*), ginger juice stir-fried Cortex Eucommiae Ulmoidis (*Du Zhong*), wine-washed Radix Angelicae Sinensis (*Dang Gui*), wine-washed Radix Dipsaci (*Xu Duan*), clam shell stir-fried Gelatinum Corii Asini (*E Jiao*), four (Ingredients) processed Rhizoma Cyperi Rotundi (*Xiang Fu*), Herba Leonuri Heterophylli (*Yi Mu Cao*), stir-fried Radix Scutellariae Baicalensis (*Huang Qin*), Pericarpium Citri Reticulatae (*Chen Pi*), Radix Ligustici Wallichii (*Chuan Xiong*), vinegar mix-fried Folium Artemisiae Argyii (*Ai Ye*), powdered Fructus Amomi (*Sha Ren*), made into pills with the flesh of Fructus Zizyphi Jujubae (*Da Zao*). Take 9-12g each time on an empty stomach washed down with rice soup.

7. *Du Zhong Wan* (from *Zheng Zhi Zhun Sheng [Patterns & Treatments Norms & Criteria]*): Ginger juice stir-fried Cortex Eucommiae Ulmoidis (*Du Zhong*), wine-soaked Radix Dipsaci (*Xu Duan*), equal amounts ground into fine powder. Mix with water and the flesh of Fructus Zizyphi Jujubae (*Da Zao*) and make into pills. Take 9g each time, washed down with rice soup.

147

8. *Liu Wei Di Huang Wan:* See Section Nine, Chapter Four.

9. *Dang Gui San:* See Section Three, Chapter Five.

10. *Huang Qin Bai Zhu Tang:* Radix Scutellariae Baicalensis (*Huang Qin*), Rhizoma Atractylodis Macrocephalae (*Bai Zhu*), Radix Angelicae Sinensis (*Dang Gui*), Radix Glycyrrhizae (*Gan Cao*)

11. *Liang Tai Yin* (from *Jing Yue Quan Shu [Jing-yue's Complete Writings]):* Uncooked Radix Rehmanniae (*Sheng Di*), Radix Albus Paeoniae Lactiflorae (*Bai Shao*), Radix Scutellariae Baicalensis (*Huang Qin*), Radix Angelicae Sinensis (*Dang Gui*), Radix Glycyrrhizae (*Gan Cao*), Fructus Citri Seu Ponciri (*Zhi Ke*), Herba Dendrobii (*Shi Hu*), Sclerotium Poriae Cocos (*Fu Ling*)

Section Seven

Edema During Pregnancy (*Ren Shen Zhong Zhang*)

If , during pregnancy, the signs of swelling and distention appear, this is called swelling and distention (or edema) during pregnancy. This was mentioned as early as the *Jin Gui Yao Lue (Essentials from the Golden Cabinet)*. In ancient dynasties, this was called by several names. These are derived from the fact that its symptoms are not all the same. Thus there are *zhi zhong*, fetal swelling, *zi man*, fetal fullness, *zi qi*, fetal qi, *cui jiao*, fragile feet, and *zhou jiao*, wrinkled feet. Superficial edema of the face and head extending to the body with short, scanty urination is called fetal swelling. Abdominal distention, fullness, and panting occurring in the 6-7th months is fetal fullness. If the knees and feet are swollen and the urination is long, this is fetal qi. If both feet are swollen and the skin is thick, this is wrinkled feet. If booth feet are swollen but the skin is thin, this is fragile feet.

Disease Causes, Disease Mechanisms

In general, the cause of this disease is water qi and damp evils stopping and accumulating. The spleen may be vacuous and not able to transport and transform water dampness. The kidneys may be vacuous and not able to disinhibit water. The fetal child with advancing months grows large and thus the qi mechanism of the viscera and bowels easily loses its regulation. Hence the transportation and movement of qi and blood are inhibited. qi becomes stagnant and dampness obstructs, etc. Any of these may result in this disease.

Disease Patterns

Spleen Vacuity

In mild cases, the pregnant woman has superficial edema spreading from her head and face to her limbs and body. The skin is a moist, white color and is bright. There is dizziness, heaviness of the head, a bland, slimy taste and sensation in the mouth, lack of strength in the four limbs, vexation and worry, restlessness, if severe, panting (*i.e.*, asthmatic breathing), short, scanty urination, and loose stools. The tongue coating is white and slimy, and the pulse image is deep and slippery. This superficial edema gradually develops from the beginning of pregnancy.

In severe cases, the pregnant woman experiences whole body superficial edema, abdominal fullness and distention which is extremely unusual, qi counterflow, restlessness, difficult, astringent urination, dizziness, heaviness of the head, a bland mouth, heart palpitations, a white, slimy tongue coating, and a vacuous, slippery pulse image. In heavy cases, extreme fatigue, threatened abortion, and even fetal death may occur.

Kidney Vacuity

The woman has been pregnant for several months. There is superficial edema of the face and limbs. The face has a dark, dull color. There are heart palpitations, shortness of breath, fear of chill by the lower extremities,

149

low back soreness, and abdominal fullness. The tongue is pale with a thin, white or glossy coating. the pulse image is fine and slow or deep and slow.

Qi Stagnation

During pregnancy, the lower limbs, low back, or lower body have superficial edema. Movement is hard and difficult. If severe, yellowish water may be discharged from between the toes. There is essence spirit depression, dizziness, and pain and distention of the head. The appetite is scant and the tongue coating is thick and slimy. The pulse is deep, wiry, and slippery.

Treatment

Spleen Vacuity

One should rectify the spleen and move water. The formula to use is *Ze Xie San* (Alisma Powder) or *Kui Zi Fu Ling San* (Abutilon & Poria Powder). If severe, one can use *Fu Ling Dao Shui Tang* (Poria Abduct Water Decoction) or *Quan Sheng Bai Shi San* (*Whole Life* Atractylodes Powder), or *Qian Jin Li Yu Tang* (*Thousand [Pieces of] Gold* Carp Decoction).

Kidney Vacuity

One should warm the kidneys and move water. The formula to use is *Zhen Wu Tang* (True Warrior Decoction) or *Shen Qi Wan* (Kidney Qi Pills).

Qi Stagnation

One should regulate the qi and move stagnation. The formula to use is *Tian Xian Teng San* (Caulis Aristolochiae Powder). If there is qi vacuity, one can use *Bu Zhong Yi Qi Tang* (Supplement the Center & Boost the Qi Decoction) plus Sclerotium Poriae Cocos (*Fu Ling*).

Explanation

1. Edema of the lower extremities is considered normal in the last trimester as long as it is unaccompanied by any other particular discomfort and as long as prenatal examination likewise reveals no other abnormalities.

2. In the treatment of this disease, it is necessary to mainly fortify the spleen and seep dampness, normalize the qi and quiet the fetus. Following the pattern, one can use the following medicinal ingredients:

A. For fortifying the spleen: Radix Panacis Ginseng (*Ren Shen*), Rhizoma Atractylodis Macrocephalae (*Bai Zhu*), Sclerotium Poriae Cocos (*Fu Ling*), Radix Glycyrrhizae (*Gan Cao*)

B. For seeping dampness: Sclerotium Poriae Cocos (*Fu Ling*), Rhizoma Alismatis (*Ze Xie*), Pericarpium Arecae Catechu (*Da Fu Pi*), Semen Abutilonis Seu Malvae (*Dong Kui Zi*), Radix Stephaniae Tetrandrae (*Fang Ji*), Sclerotium Polypori Umbellati (*Zhu Ling*), uncooked Cortex Rhizomatis Zingiberis (*Sheng Jiang Pi*), Cortex Radicis Mori Albi (*Sang Bai Pi*)

C. For normalizing the qi: Caulis Aristolochiae Debilis (*Tian Xian Teng*), Caulis Perillae Frutescentis (*Su Gen*), Rhizoma Cyperi Rotundi (*Xiang Fu*), Radix Linderae Strychnifoliae (*Wu Yao*), Radix Saussureae Seu Vladimiriae (*Mu Xiang*), Fructus Amomi (*Sha Ren*), Fructus Citri Seu Ponciri (*Zhi Ke*), Pericarpium Citri Reticulatae (*Chen Pi*), Lignum Dalbergiae Odoriferae (*Jiang Xiang*)

D. For quieting the fetus: Ramus Loranthi Seu Visci (*Sang Ji Sheng*), Radix Scutellariae Baicalensis (*Huang Qin*), Rhizoma Atractylodis Macrocephalae (*Bai Zhu*), Cortex Eucommiae Ulmoidis (*Du Zhong*)

E. For nourishing the blood: Radix Angelicae Sinensis (*Dang Gui*), Radix Albus Paeoniae Lactiflorae (*Bai Shao*)

3. Clinically, *Fu Ling Dao Shui Tang* (Poria Abduct Water Decoction) is the most frequently used formula for the treatment of edema during

151

pregnancy. As soon as the swelling subsides and dampness is eliminated, *Liu Jun Zi Tang* (Six Gentlemen Decoction) should be used to regulate and rectify and thus prevent relapse. *Qian Jin Li Yu Tang* (*Thousand [Pieces of] Gold* Carp Decoction) treats fetal water swelling and fullness due to spleen vacuity with simultaneous blood vacuity with good results. If there is qi stagnation or heavy dampness, it is not appropriate to use this.

4. In this disease, proper nursing is also very important. Food and drink should regularly be low salt and clear and bland. Frequent urine tests and blood pressure readings are also recommended. Albuminuria, hypertension, and superficial edema are commonly seen symptoms of poisoning during pregnancy. Therefore, prompt treatment should be given to prevent the onset of fetal epilepsy or eclampsia gravidarum.

Appended Formulas

1. *Ze Xie San (*from *Chan Bao [Birthing Treasure]):* Rhizoma Alismatis (*Ze Xie*), stir-fried Cortex Radicis Mori Albi (*Sang Bai Pi*), Caulis Akebiae Mutong (*Mu Tong*), stir-fried Fructus Citri Seu Ponciri (*Zhi Ke*), Semen Arecae Catechu (*Bing Lang*), Sclerotium Rubrum Poriae Cocos (*Chi Fu Ling*)

2. *Kui Zi Fu Ling San (*from *Jin Gui Yao Lue [Essentials from the Golden Cabinet]):* Semen Abutilonis Seu Malvae (*Dong Kui Zi*), Sclerotium Poriae Cocos (*Fu Ling*). Grind into powder. Take 6g each time, 3 times per day. Disinhibition of the urination results in cure.

3. *Fu Ling Dao Shui Tang (*from *Yi Zong Jin Jian (Golden Mirror of Ancestral Medicine]):* Radix Saussureae Seu Vladimiriae (*Mu Xiang*), Fructus Chaenomelis Lagenariae (*Mu Gua*), Semen Arecae Catechu (*Bing Lang*), Pericarpium Arecae Catechu (*Da Fu Pi*), Rhizoma Atractylodis Macrocephalae (*Bai Zhu*), Sclerotium Polypori Umbellati (*Zhu Ling*), Rhizoma Alismatis (*Ze Xie*), Cortex Radicis Mori Albi (*Sang Bai Pi*), Fructus Amomi (*Sha Ren*), Folium Perillae Frutescentis (*Su Ye*), Pericarpium Citri Reticulatae (*Chen Pi*)

4. *Quan Sheng Bai Zhu San* (from *Quan Sheng Zhi Mi Fang [Whole Life Pointing Out Confusion Formulas]):* Pericarpium Arecae Catechu (*Da Fu Pi*), Rhizoma Atractylodis Macrocephalae (*Bai Zhu*), uncooked Cortex Rhizomatis Zingiberis (*Sheng Jiang Pi*), Sclerotium Poriae Cocos (*Fu Ling*), Exocarpium Citri Grandis (*Ju Pi*)

5. *Qian Jin Li Yu Tang* (from *Qian Jin Fang [Formulas {Worth a} Thousand {Pieces of} Gold]):* Rhizoma Atractylodis Macrocephalae (*Bai Zhu*), Sclerotium Poriae Cocos (*Fu Ling*), Radix Angelicae Sinensis (*Dang Gui*), Radix Albus Paeoniae Lactiflorae (*Bai Shao*). Grind the above medicinals into powder. Take 12g and boil these together with 2 cups of soup from a medium-sized carp prepared as one typically would for home use. Add 7 slices of uncooked Rhizoma Zingiberis (*Sheng Jiang*) and a small amount of Pericarpium Citri Reticulatae (*Chen Pi*) and cook until this soup is reduced to about 70% of its original volume by boiling. Then drink the broth.

6. *Zhen Wu Tang* (from *Shang Han Lun [Treatise in Damage Due to Cold]):* Sclerotium Poriae Cocos (*Fu Ling*), Radix Albus Paeoniae Lactiflorae (*Bai Shao*), Rhizoma Atractylodis Macrocephalae (*Bai Zhu*), uncooked Rhizoma Zingiberis (*Sheng Jiang*), Radix Lateralis Praeparatus Aconiti Carmichaeli (*Fu Zi*)

7. *Shen Qi Wan* (from *Jin Gui Yao Lue [Essentials from the Golden Cabinet]):* Dry Radix Rehmanniae (*Gan di Huang*), Radix Dioscoreae Oppositae (*Shan Yao*), Fructus Corni Officinalis (*Shan Zhu Yu*), Sclerotium Poriae Cocos (*Fu Ling*), Cortex Radicis Moutan (*Dan Pi*), Ramulus Cinnamomi (*Gui Zhi*), Rhizoma Alismatis (*Ze Xie*), Radix Lateralis Praeparata Aconiti Carmichaeli (*Fu Zi*)

8. *Tian Xian Teng San* (from *Fu Ren Da Quan Liang Fang [A Great, Complete {Collection of} Fine Formulas for Women]):* Caulis Aristolochiae Debilis (*Tian Xian Teng*), Rhizoma Cyperi Rotundi (*Xiang Fu*), Pericarpium Citri Reticulatae (*Chen Pi*), Radix Glycyrrhizae (*Gan Cao*), Radix Linderae Strychnifoliae (*Wu Yao*), uncooked Rhizoma Zingiberis

(*Sheng Jiang*), Fructus Chaenomelis Lagenariae (*Mu Gua*), Folium Perillae Frutescentis (*Su Ye*)

9. *Bu Zhong Yi Qi Tang:* See Section One, Chapter Four.

Section Eight

Fetal Epilepsy (*Zi Xian*)

In the latter stage of pregnancy or just prior to or just after delivery, there may be repeated attacks of a series of symptoms, such as vertigo, dizziness, fainting, tremors and contraction of the limbs, lockjaw, staring eyes, and lack of consciousness of human affairs. These symptoms are called *zi xian*, fetal epilepsy (*i.e.*, eclampsia). Fetal epilepsy is one of the most serious diseases occurring during pregnancy. It commonly threatens the life destiny of both the mother and infant. Therefore, in clinical practice, it is important that it be given timely preventive treatment.

Disease Causes, Disease Mechanisms

The disease mechanisms causing the onset of fetal epilepsy are the pregnant woman's constitutional yin vacuity and blood vacuity with yang qi tending to be hyperactive. After conception, blood nourishes the fetal origin. If yin blood become deficient, vacuity fire may blaze. If there is yin vacuity and blood deficiency, blood does not nourish the sinews which thus leads to contracture of the sinew vessels. Phlegm turbidity may join and blaze, harassing above the clear portals. It may also be due to blood heat contracting wind and leading to its arising.

Disease Patterns

Blood Heat Contracting Wind

In the latter stage of pregnancy, there is sudden fainting, tremors and contractions of the four limbs, lockjaw, clouded spirit, a flushed red facial

154

complexion, and possible epigastric pain, vomiting, or constipation before an attack. The tongue is red, and the pulse is wiry, slippery, and rapid.

Blood Vacuity Wind Heat

In the latter stage of pregnancy, there is a somber white facial complexion, headache, vertigo, heart palpitations, shortness of breath, spiritual fatigue, slack limbs, occasional red cheeks, fetal stirring, abdominal pain, dry stools, a red tongue with a scant coating, and a wiry, fine, rapid pulse. At the time of an attack, there is vertigo, dizziness, abrupt fainting, lockjaw, cramping in the limbs, and rigidity of the neck.

Qi Depression, Phlegm Stagnation

The pregnant woman's body is fat and obese or there may be pronounced superficial edema. The body is cold and there is chest and epigastric fullness and oppression, vomiting of phlegm drool, and essence spirit fatigue. The tongue coating is white and slimy, and the pulse image is wiry and slippery. At the time of attack, there is sudden fainting and dizziness, vomiting of phlegm drool, tremor and contraction of the limbs, and loss of consciousness of human affairs.

Treatment

Blood Heat Contracting Wind

One should clear heat and stabilize wind. The formula to use is *Ling Yang Jiao San* (Antelope Horn Powder) and *Gou Teng Tang* (Uncaria Decoction). If there is qi vacuity, add Radix Panacis Ginseng (*Ren Shen*). If there is spleen vacuity, Rhizoma Atractylodis Macrocephalae (*Bai Zhu*). And if there is wind tetany, add Succus Bambusae (*Zhu Li*, Concretio Silicae Bambusae (*Tian Zhu Huang*), and Bulbus Fritillariae (*Bei Mu*).

Blood Vacuity Wind Heat

One should nourish the blood and stabilize wind. The formula to use is *Jia Wei Xi Jiao Di Huang Tang* (Added Flavors Rhinoceros Horn & Rehmannia Decoction). If qi and blood are both vacuous, one can use *Ba Zhen Tang* (Eight Pearls Decoction) plus Ramulus Uncariae Cum Uncis (*Gou Teng*), Flos Chrysanthemi Morifolii (*Ju Hua*), and Fructus Ligustri Lucidi (*Nu Zhen Zi*).

Qi Depression, Phlegm Stagnation

One should wash away phlegm and transform stagnation, expel wind and scatter cold. the formula to use is *Ge Gen Tang* (Pueraria Decoction). If there is phlegm heat, one can remove Cortex Cinnamomi (*Rou Gui*) and add Succus Bambusae (*Zhu Li*) and processed Rhizoma Pinelliae Ternatae (*Ban Xia*).

Explanation

1. Efforts should be made to differentiate fetal epilepsy from wind stroke, tetanus, epilepsy, brain disease, and medicinal poisoning. Thus, in clinical practice, intensive inquiry is always required so as to assure a correct diagnosis. It is not alright to treat all these as one disease.

2. It is often noted that, in varying degrees, headache and dizziness, loss of sleep and heart vexation, abdominal distention and nausea, and superficial edema and scanty urination may precede an attack of fetal epilepsy. This is called pre-fetal epilepsy (*i.e.*, pre-eclampsia) clinically. In fact, in order to control fetal epilepsy attacks, it is important to pay attention to the early treatment of pre-fetal epilepsy.

3. Those who have water swelling and high blood pressure are instructed to rest in bed and to eat a low salt diet.

4. No matter whether this disease occurs during pregnancy or at delivery, treatment should mainly nourish the blood and extinguish wind, level the

liver and transform phlegm. If it occurs after delivery, one should mainly greatly supplement the qi and blood.

5. During an attack, in order to prevent injury to the tongue by biting, one can place a wooden tongue depressor wrapped with gauze in the patient's mouth.

6. In those with excessive phlegm, one can use Succus Bambusae (*Zhu Li*) and several drops of ginger juice (*Jiang Ye*) taken warm. This gets good results in transforming phlegm.

7. If Cornu Antelopis (*Ling Yang Jiao*) is scarce and prohibitively expensive (not mention endangered ecologically), one can use Carapax Eretmochelydis (*Tai Mao*) instead.

Appended Formulas

1. *Ling Yang Jiao San* (from *Pu Ji Ben Shi Fang [Formulas of Universal Benefit from My Practice])*: Cornu Antelopis (*Ling Yang Jiao*), Radix Angelicae Pubescentis (*Du Huo*), stir-fried Semen Zizyphi Spinosae (*Zao Ren*), Cortex Radicis Acanthopanacis (*Wu Jia Pi*), stir-fried Semen Coicis Lachryma-jobi (*Mi Ren*), Radix Ledebouriellae Sesloidis (*Fang Feng*), wine(-processed) Radix Angelicae Sinensis (*Dang Gui*), Radix Ligustici Wallichii (*Chuan Xiong*), Sclerotium Pararadicis Poriae Cocos (*Fu Shen*), Semen Pruni Armeniacae (*Xing Ren*), Radix Saussureae Seu Vladimiriae (*Mu Xiang*), Radix Glycyrrhizae (*Gan Cao*), uncooked Rhizoma Zingiberis (*Sheng Jiang*)

2. *Gou Teng Tang* (from *Fu Ren Da Quan Liang Fang [A Great, Complete {Collection of} Fine Formulas for Women])*: Ramulus Uncariae Cum Uncis (*Gou Teng*), Radix Angelicae Sinensis (*Dang Gui*), Sclerotium Pararadicis Poriae Cocos (*Fu Shen*), Radix Panacis Ginseng (*Ren Shen*), Exocarpium Citri Grandis (*Ju Pi*), Ramus Loranthi Seu Visci (*Sang Ji Sheng*)

3. *Jia Wei Xi Jiao Di Huang Tang* (from *Zhong Guo Fu Ke Bing Xue [The Study of Gynecological Diseases in China])*: Cornu Rhinocerotis (*Xi Jiao*;

substitute Cornu Bubali [*Shui Niu Jiao*]), uncooked Radix Rehmanniae (*Sheng Di*), Radix Albus Paeoniae Lactiflorae (*Bai Shao*), stir-fried Fructus Immaturus Citri Seu Ponciri (*Zhi Ke*), Ramulus Uncariae Cum Uncis (*Gou Teng*), Sclerotium Pararadicis Poriae Cocos (*Fu Shen*), Pericarpium Citri Reticulatae (*Chen Pi*), Radix Angelicae Sinensis (*Dang Gui*), Tuber Ophiopogonis Japonicae (*Mai Dong*), stir-fried Cortex Magnoliae Officinalis (*Hou Po*)

4. *Ba Zhen Tang:* See Section Two, Chapter Five.

5. *Ge Gen Tang (*from *Wai Tai Mi Yao [Secret Essentials from an External Desk]):* Bulbus Fritillariae (*Bei Mu*), Radix Puerariae (*Ge Gen*), Cortex Radicis Moutan (*Dan Pi*), Radix Stephaniae Tetrandrae (*Fang Ji*), Radix Ledebouriellae Sesloidis (*Fang Feng*), Radix Angelicae Sinensis (*Dang Gui*), Radix Ligustici Wallichii (*Chuan Xiong*), Cortex Cinnamomi (*Rou Gui*), Sclerotium Poriae Cocos (*Fu Ling*), Rhizoma Alismatis (*Ze Xie*), Radix Angelicae Pubescentis (*Du Huo*), Gypsum Fibrosum (*Shi Gao*), Radix Panacis Ginseng (*Ren Shen*), Radix Glycyrrhizae (*Gan Cao*)

Section Nine

Fetal Pressure (*Zhuan Bao*) (also know as Non-free-flowing Urination During Pregnancy [*Ren Shen Xiao Bian Bu Tong*])

During pregnancy, if the urination is not free-flowing and, if severe, there is lower abdominal distention, tension, aching, and pain, this is what the *Jin Gui Yao Lue (Essentials from the Golden Cabinet)* calls fetal pressure (literally turned uterus). Later, the *Zhu Bing Yuan Hou Lun (Treatise on the Origins & Symptoms of Various Diseases)* refers to this as urination during pregnancy not free-flowing.

Disease Causes, Disease Mechanisms

Clinically, in this disease, repletion and vacuity are not the same. Vacuity means mainly qi vacuity and kidney vacuity. The fetal qi sags downward and presses upon the bladder. This results in the bladder being inhibited and the water passageways are not free-flowing. Thus the urine does not discharge by itself. Repletion is mostly duet to damp heat pouring downward to the bladder. Thus there is heat depression and qi binding and the water passageways are inhibited. It is also possible that as the fetus grows, this puts pressure on the bladder. Its qi mechanism is thus inhibited.

Disease Patterns

Qi Vacuity

Urination during pregnancy dribbles by the drop and is not free-flowing. It may also be frequent, numerous, and scanty. The facial complexion is somber white, and there are heart palpitations, shortness of breath, dizziness, lack of strength, a pale tongue with a thin, white coating, and a vacuous, fine, slippery pulse.

Kidney Vacuity

Urination during pregnancy dribbles by the drop and is not free-flowing. There is lower abdominal inflation and distention, superficial edema of the face and limbs, a dark, dull facial complexion, bodily fatigue and lack of strength, dizziness, fear of chill, low back and knee soreness and weakness, and loose stools. The tongue is pale and lusterless. The coating is thin, white, and slimy. The pulse image is deep and slow or deep, slippery, and forceless.

Damp Heat

The urination is inhibited or yellowish red, short and scanty. here is lower abdominal distention and pain, heart vexation, internal heat, heaviness of the head and clouding, a bitter taste in the mouth, dry, bound stools or possible diarrhea or non-crisp stools. The tongue is red with a thin, yellow or white, slimy coating. the pulse image is slippery and rapid.

Qi Stagnation

During the 7-8th months of pregnancy, there is sudden non-free flow of urination, lower abdominal distention, tension, aching, and pain, heart vexation, chest oppression, a thin, slimy tongue coating, and a deep, wiry pulse.

Treatment

Qi Vacuity

One should supplement the qi, upbear and lift. The formula to use is *Bu Zhong Yi Qi Tang* (Supplement the Center & Boost the Qi Decoction). If qi and blood are both vacuous, one can use *Ba Zhen Tang* (Eight Pearls Decoction) or *Ju Tai Si Wu Tang* (Lift the Fetus Four Materials Decoction).

Kidney Vacuity

One should supplement the kidneys and warm yang, transform qi and move water. The formula to use is *Jin Gui Shen Qi Wan* (Golden Cabinet Kidney Qi Pills).

Damp Heat

One should clear heat and eliminate dampness. The formula to use is *Quan Sheng Fu Ling San* (*Whole Life* Poria Powder) or *Dong Kui Zi San* (Abutilon Pills). If heat bind is severe, use *Dang Gui Bei Mu Ku Sheng Wan* (Dang Gui, Fritillaria & Sophora Pills).

Qi Stagnation

One should course the qi and transform stagnation. The formula to use is *Fen Qi Yin* (Divide the Qi Drink).

Explanation

1. This disease is mostly due to central qi vacuity weakness. Qi vacuity does not gather and the fetal origin descends putting pressure on the bladder. Treatment methods should mainly supplement the qi, upbear and raise. However, before complications due to vacuity, heat and stagnation are completely treated, it is not appropriate to overuse coursing and abduction.

2. Fetal pressure is an acute condition during pregnancy. Therefore, it may be necessary to augment treatment via catheterization or surgery.

Appended Formulas

1. *Bu Zhong Yi Qi Tang:* See Section One, Chapter Four.

2. *Ba Zhen Tang:* See Section Two, Chapter Five.

3. *Ju Tai Si Wu Tang (*from *Yi Zong Jin Jian [Golden Mirror of Ancestral Medicine]):* Radix Angelicae Sinensis (*Dang Gui*), prepared Radix Rehmanniae (*Shu Di*), Radix Ligustici Wallichii (*Chuan Xiong*), Radix Panacis Ginseng (*Ren Shen*), Rhizoma Atractylodis Macrocephalae (*Bai Zhu*), Pericarpium Citri Reticulatae (*Chen Pi*), Rhizoma Cimicifugae (*Sheng Ma*), Radix Glycyrrhizae (*Gan Cao*)

4. *Jin Gui Shen Qi Wan (*from *Jin Gui Yao Lue [Essentials from the Golden Cabinet]):* Dry Radix Rehmanniae (*Gan Di Huang*), Radix Dioscoreae Oppositae (*Shan Yao*), Fructus Corni Officinalis (*Shan Zhu Yu*), Rhizoma Alismatis (*Ze Xie*), Cortex Radicis Moutan (*Dan Pi*), Ramulus Cinnamomi

161

(*Gui Zhi*), Radix Lateralis Praeparatus Aconiti Carmichaeli Praeparati (*Fu Zi*), Sclerotium Poriae Cocos (*Fu Ling*)

5. *Quan Sheng Fu Ling San* (from *Jian Yi Fang [Simple, Easy Formulas]*): Sclerotium Rubrum Poriae Cocos (*Chi Fu Ling*), Semen Abutilonis Seu Malvae (*Dong Kui Zi*), equal amounts. Grind these into a fine powder and take 15g each time, 2 times per day.

6. *Dong Kui Zi San* (from *Ji Yin Gang Mu [Detailed Outline of Yin]*): Semen Abutilonis Seu Malvae (*Dong Kui Zi*), stir-fried Fructus Gardeniae Jasminoidis (*Zhi Zi*), Talcum (*Hua Shi*), Caulis Akebiae Mutong (*Mu Tong*)

7. *Dang Gui Bei Mu Ku Shen Wan* (from *Jin Gui Yao Lue [Essentials from the Golden Cabinet]*): Radix Angelicae Sinensis (*Dang Gui*), Bulbus Fritillariae (*Bei Mu*), Radix Sophorae Flavescentis (*Ku Shen*), equal amounts. Grind these into a fine powder and make into pills the size of red beans with honey. Take 3-10 pills each time.

8. *Fen Qi Yin* (from *Fu Ren Da Quan Liang Fang [A Great, Complete {Collection of} Fine Formulas for Women]*): Pericarpium Citri Reticulatae (*Chen Pi*), Sclerotium Poriae Cocos (*Fu Ling*), Rhizoma Pinelliae Ternatae (*Ban Xia*), Radix Platycodi Grandiflori (*Jie Geng*), Pericarpium Arecae Catechu (*Da Fu Pi*), Caulis Perillae Frutescentis (*Su Gen*), Fructus Citri Seu Ponciri (*Zhi Ke*), Rhizoma Atractylodis Macrocephalae (*Bai Zhu*), Fructus Gardeniae Jasminoidis (*Shan Zhi*), Radix Glycyrrhizae (*Gan Cao*)

9. A surgical treatment method of Zhu Dan-xi: After sterilizing the hands, the attending midwife tries to elevate the fetus by stretching out her hands into the vagina to relieve the emergency (*i.e.* anuria). This method can be followed by taking supplementing and boosting medicinals. After taking the medicinals, the patient should try to induce vomiting by putting their fingers down their throat. After vomiting, take more medicinals. Repeat 3-4 times and the fetus will lifted and urination will automatically be disinhibited.

Chapter Seven

Postpartum Diseases (*Chan Hou Bing*)

Postpartum diseases mainly refer to diseases whose onset occurs during the puerperium (literally, the birth mat period). Thus they are called after birth or postpartum diseases. During this entire period, due to wounds and damage and hemorrhage sustained during stagnant parturition and excessive use of force during birthing, the birthing woman's original qi may have sustained detriment. Thus her power of resistance may be reduced and weak, and this easily leads to the arising of disease. The main causes leading to the arising of postpartum diseases are: 1) detriment and damage to the *chong* and *ren*, excessive loss of blood, and perished blood damaging fluids; 2) cold congelation/qi stagnation, static blood internally obstructing; and 3) external invasion by the six environmental excesses or damage due to food and drink or bedroom taxation, any of which may lead to postpartum disease. Commonly seen postpartum diseases include abdominal pain, a postpartum lochia which does not descend, a lochia which does not cease, postpartum blood dizziness, postpartum fever, postpartum tetany, postpartum difficult defecation, and postpartum scanty lactation.

In addition to the four examinations, the eight principles, and pattern discrimination, other factors should also be taken into account when diagnosing each individual case, such as the three examinations (*san shen*): 1) examination of the lochia and abdominal pain in order to discriminate repletion and vacuity in disease; 2) examination of whether the stools are free-flowing or not free-flowing in order to assess the exuberance and debility of fluids and humors; and 3) examination to see if the milk moves or does not move and whether food and drink are excessive or scanty in order to determine if the stomach qi is strong or weak. Only when these three examinations are combined with the signs and symptoms, pulse image, and tongue and tongue coating is one able to correctly diagnose postpartum diseases.

In the treatment of postpartum diseases, there are some who advocate mainly supplementing vacuity, there are some who advocate mainly transforming stasis, and these methods are not each the same. Postpartum diseases may be vacuous or replete and it is necessary to analyze the nature of the disease carefully integrated with the fact that postpartum the is a lot of vacuity and a lot of stasis. Likewise, one must also take into consideration the qi and blood as well as the condition of the spleen and stomach. Opening depression must not consume and scatter. Transforming phlegm should not attack and dispel. When dispersing food, one must simultaneously support the spleen. In clearing heat, one must not use too many bitter, cold medicinals. When resolving the exterior, do not overuse emitting and scattering. When dispelling cold, do not overuse acrid, hot medicinals. In other words, the guiding principles should be to supplement without causing stagnation evils and to attack evils without damaging the righteous qi. One should conduct treatment on the basis of pattern discrimination.

Section One

Postpartum Abdominal Pain (*Chan Hou Fu Tong*)

Postpartum abdominal pain refers to the occurrence of lower abdominal aching and pain in birthing women after parturition. This is called postpartum abdominal pain or baby pillow pain (*er zhen tong*). It may also be called static lump pain (*yu kuai tong*).

Disease Causes, Disease Mechanisms

The most commonly seen causes of postpartum abdominal pain are static blood abdominal pain, blood vacuity abdominal pain, and vacuity cold abdominal pain, these three types. Static blood abdominal pain is due to postpartum blood stasis being retained and stagnating which is not expelled. Blood vacuity abdominal pain is due to excessive blood having been expelled after delivery. Thus the *bao mai* is not nourished. Vacuity cold abdominal pain is due to excessive blood having been expelled allowing for the contraction of wind cold evils lodging in the uterus. As the *Yi Zong Jin Jian (The Golden Mirror of Ancestral Medicine)* says:

> Postpartum abdominal pain — if there is excessive loss of blood, there will be pain. Because there is blood vacuity, thus there is pain. If the lochia expelled is scanty and static blood congests and stagnates, there will be pain. This then produces aching and pain. If wind evils take advantage of vacuity and enter the uterus causing pain, one must see chilly pain and a strong body.

This is the differential diagnosis of postpartum abdominal pain.

Disease Patterns

Static Blood Abdominal Pain

The postpartum lochia is scanty of stops prematurely. There is sudden lower abdominal aching and pain which is spasmodic in nature. When there is pain, lumps attack and push or there appear hardness and fullness. There is no desire for pressure. The stools may be difficult, but the urination is uninhibited. The tongue is purple and dark, and the pulse image is deep, wiry, choppy, and has force.

Blood Vacuity Abdominal Pain

Postpartum the blood expelled is excessive. Abdominal pain likes pressure. The pain is continuous and mild and there are no lumps attacking and pushing. There is dizziness, vertigo, slight fever, night sweats, and bodily fatigue. The tongue is pale with a thin, white coating, and the pulse is fine and relaxed (*i.e.,* retarded).

Vacuity Cold Abdominal Pain

There is pain in the lower abdomen pain radiating to the navel. This pain tends to be continuous and likes pressure or likes hot applications. The

165

lochia is scanty and there is inversion chill of the four limbs or fear of cold, a pale white facial complexion, essence spirit fatigue, a thin, white tongue coating, and a vacuous, slow pulse.

Treatment

Static Blood Abdominal Pain

One should dispel stasis and engender the new. If mild, the formula to use is *Shi Xiao San* (Sudden Smile Powder), *Yan Hu Suo San* (Corydalis Powder), or *Jia Wei Sheng Hua Tang* (Added Flavors Engendering & Transforming Decoction). If heavy and there is simultaneous vexation and agitation, fever, delirious speech, and a vacuous pulse, one can use *Da Cheng Qi Tang* (Major Order the Qi Decoction).

Blood Vacuity Abdominal Pain

One should warm and nourish the qi and blood. The formula to use is *Dang Gui Jian Zhong Tang* (Dang Gui Fortify the Center Decoction), *Si Wu Tang Jia Pao Jiang Shen Zhu* (Four Materials Decoction plus Blast-fried Ginger, Ginseng & Atractylodes), or *Chang Ning Tang* (Intestines Quieting Decoction).

Vacuity Cold Abdominal Pain

One should warm the channels and nourish the blood. The formula to use is *Dang Gui Sheng Jiang Yang Rou Tang* (Dang Gui, Fresh Ginger & Lamb Decoction) or *Xiang Gui San* (Fragrant Cinnamon Powder). If there is simultaneous blood stasis, *Sheng Hua Tang* (Engendering & Transforming Decoction) is appropriate.

Explanation

1. Postpartum abdominal pain mostly develops 1-2 days after delivery due to static blood retained internally or to invasion of cold and cool around the

time of delivery. Except during the midsummer when heat flares, *Sheng Hua Tang* (Transforming & Engendering Decoction) is the correct treatment, plus Herba Lycopi Lucidi (*Ze Lan*), Folium Artemisiae Argyii (*Ai Ye*), Herba Leonuri Heterophylli (*Yi Mu Cao*), etc., following the pattern. In addition, a soup made from the flesh of Fructus Crataegi (*Shan Zha*) taken orally treats child pillow pain with good results. Besides being able to disperse food and open the stomach, it is equally able to harmonize the blood and disperse stasis.

2. Postpartum abdominal pain is not often categorized as only vacuity. For example, pain which likes pressure occurring several days after delivery is mostly categorized as blood vacuity and qi stagnation. For its treatment, one should use nourishing the blood medicinals plus stir-fried Fructus Meliae Toosendan (*Chuan Lian Zi*) and Semen Citri Reticulatae (*Ju He*). When vacuity and repletion occur together, based on the presenting pattern, one should make careful analysis.

Appended Formulas

1. *Shi Xiao San:* See Section Ten, Chapter Four.

2. *Yan Hu Suo San (*from *Ji Yin Gang Mu [Detailed Outline of Yin]):* Rhizoma Corydalis Yanhusuo (*Yan Hu Suo*), Cortex Cinnamomi (*Gui Xin*), Radix Angelicae Sinensis (*Dang Gui*)

3. *Jia Wei Sheng Hua Tang (*from *Fu Qing Zhu Nu Ke [Fu Qing-zhu's Gynecology]):* Radix Angelicae Sinensis (*Dang Gui*), Radix Ligustici Wallichii (*Chuan Xiong*), uncooked Rhizoma Zingiberis (*Sheng Jiang*), Semen Pruni Persicae (*Tao Ren*), Herba Lycopi Lucidi (*Ze Lan*), Folium Artemisiae Argyii (*Ai Ye*), Herba Leonuri Heterophylli (*Yi Mu Cao*)

4. *Da Cheng Qi Tang (*from *Shang Han Lun [Treatise on Damage Due to Cold]):* Radix Et Rhizoma Rhei (*Da Huang*), Mirabilitum (*Mang Xiao*), Cortex Magnoliae Officinalis (*Hou Po*), Fructus Immaturus Citri Seu Ponciri (*Zhi Shi*)

5. *Dang Gui Jian Zhong Tang* (from *Qian Jin Yao Fang [Formulas {Worth} a Thousand {Pieces of} Gold]*): Radix Angelicae Sinensis (*Dang Gui*), stir-fried Radix Albus Paeoniae Lactiflorae (*Bai Shao*), Ramulus Cinnamomi (*Gui Zhi*), mix-fried Radix Glycyrrhizae (*Zhi Gan Cao*), uncooked Rhizoma Zingiberis (*Sheng Jiang*), Fructus Zizyphi Jujubae (*Da Zao*), Maltose (*Yi Tang*)

6. *Si Wu Tang Jia Pao Jiang Shen Zhu:* Radix Angelicae Sinensis (*Dang Gui*), Radix Ligustici Wallichii (*Chuan Xiong*), stir-fried Radix Albus Paeoniae Lactiflorae (*Bai Shao*), prepared Radix Rehmanniae (*Shu Di*), blast-fried Rhizoma Zingiberis (*Pao Jiang*), Radix Panacis Ginseng (*Ren Shen*), Rhizoma Atractylodis Macrocephalae (*Bai Zhu*)

7. *Chang Ning Tang* (from *Fu Qing Zhu Nu Ke [Fu Qing-zhu's Gynecology]*): Wine-washed Radix Angelicae Sinensis (*Dang Gui*), prepared Radix Rehmanniae (*Shu Di*), Radix Panacis Ginseng (*Ren Shen*), Tuber Ophiopogonis Japonicae (*Mai Dong*), powdered clam shell stir-fried Gelatinum Corii Asini (*E Jiao*), stir-fried Radix Dioscoreae Oppositae (*Shan Yao*), Radix Dipsaci (*Xu Duan*), Radix Glycyrrhizae (*Gan Cao*), Cortex Cinnamomi (*Rou Gui*)

8. *Dang Gui Sheng Jiang Yang Rou Tang* (from *Jin Gui Yao Lue [Essentials from the Golden Cabinet]*): Lamb (*Yang Rou*), Radix Angelicae Sinensis (*Dang Gui*), Radix Ligustici Wallichii (*Chuan Xiong*), uncooked Rhizoma Zingiberis (*Sheng Jiang*). Decocted with wine (*Jiu*), Bulbus Allii Fistulosi (*Cong*), and salt (*Yan*) or with Radix Panacis Ginseng (*Ren Shen*) and Rhizoma Atractylodis Macrocephalae (*Bai Zhu*).

9. *Xiang Gui San* (from *Zheng Zhi Zhun Sheng [Patterns & Treatments Norms & Restrictions]*): Radix Angelicae Sinensis (*Dang Gui*), Radix Ligustici Wallichii (*Chuan Xiong*), Cortex Cinnamomi (*Rou Gui*). Decocted with a little infant's urine and wine and taken warm.

10. *Sheng Hua Tang:* See Section Five, Chapter Six.

Section Two

Postpartum Lochia Is Not Precipitated (*Chan Hou E Lu Bu Xia*)

After the child has been born, the residual blood and amniotic fluid retained in the uterus are called the lochia. Postpartum, the lochia should be discharged outside the body. If it stops, is retained, and is not precipitated or if it is precipitated but scantily, this is called *e lu bu xia* or lochia which is not precipitated.

Disease Causes, Disease Mechanisms

The disease causes of lochia which is not precipitated typically can be divided into the two types of vacuity and repletion. Vacuity is mostly due to excessive expulsion of blood during delivery or habitual blood deficiency on the part of the birthing woman. Since there is no blood, it is not precpitated. Repletion is due to invasion during delivery by wind chill. Qi and blood congeal and stagnate and the channels and vessels suffer obstruction. Thus the lochia is not precipitated.

Disease Patterns

Blood Stasis

There is lower abdominal chilly pain, sagging and hardness with lumps that refuse pressure, bodily cold, chilled limbs, possible vomiting and no eating, a dark tongue with a thin, white coating, and a wiry, choppy pulse.

Blood Deficiency

The lochia does not descend. There is a somber white or sallow yellow facial complexion, dizziness, blurred vision, tinnitus, heart palpitations, essence spirit fatigue, a low voice, possible tidal fever, empty pain in the

169

abdominal region which feels soft, a pale white tongue, and a vacuous, fine pulse.

Treatment

Blood Stasis

For cold congelation blood stasis with lower abdominal hardness and pain, the formula to use is *Sheng Hua Tang* (Engendering & Transforming Decoction), *Shi Xiao San* (Sudden Smile Powder). For qi stagnation and blood congelation, the formula to use is *Hua Rui Shi San* (Ophicalcitum Powder).

Blood Deficiency

For blood vacuity with fever, the formula to use is *Dang Gui Bu Xue Tang* (Dang Gui Supplement the Blood Decoction). If there is taxation damage vacuity detriment, the formula to use is *Si Wu Tang Jia Pao Jiang* (Four Materials Decoction plus Blast-fried Ginger). For abdominal pain which likes pressure, the formula to use is *Si Wu Tang Jia Pao Jiang Shen Zhu* (Four Materials Decoction plus Blast-fried Ginger, Ginseng & Atractylodes). For postpartum qi and blood dual vacuity, the formula to use is *Sheng Yu Tang* (Sage-like Healing Decoction).

Explanation

Being a normal physiological excretion, a certain amount of lochia should be discharged. If too little is discharged or discharged unsmoothly, this may be accompanied by abdominal region pain and distention. This is a pathological condition, and the corresponding treatment used is the quickening the blood and transforming stasis methods. If there is no apparent pain or distention, despite the fact that the lochia is not excessive, it is not appropriate to use blood-breaking medicinals which may make the situation worse, necessarily causing detriment and damage to the two vessels of the *chong* and *ren* combined with the production of flooding and desertion.

Postpartum there are the three surgings or *san chong*. Vanquished blood may surge into the heart (*chong xin*), leading to mania and withdrawal. If severe, one may climb up on top of high walls or their house. Surging into the lungs (*chong fei*) leads to redness of the face, panting counterflow as if on the verge of death. Surging into the stomach (*chong wei*) leads to chest oppression, vomiting, nausea, abdominal fullness, distention, and pain. These three patterns are all due to a postpartum lochia which is not precipitated. Therefore, in the case of postpartum lochia which is not precipitated, first one must determine vacuity and repletion based upon whether or not there is abdominal region pain and distention and whether one refuses or likes pressure. Abdominal region pain and distention which refuses pressure is repletion. If the abdomen has no pain and likes pressure, this is vacuity. If categorized as vacuity, do not hasten to dispel stasis. If categorized as repletion, the movement of stasis is necessarily an emergency situation. The key to the treatment of postpartum lochia which is not precipitated lies in discriminating clearly vacuity and repletion and basing one's treatment on this analysis.

Appended Formulas

1. *Sheng Hua Tang:* See Section Five, Chapter Six.

2. *Shi Xiao San:* See Section Ten, Chapter Four.

3. *Hua Rui Shi San (*from *Tai Ping Hui Min He Ji Ju Fang [Tai Ping Imperial Grace Formulary]):* Powder Ophicalcitum (*Hua Rui Shi*) and take washed down with 1 teacup of infant's urine.

4. *Dang Gui Bu Xue Tang (*from *Wei Sheng Bao Jian [Precious Mirror for Defending Life]):* Wine stir-fried Radix Angelicae Sinensis (*Dang Gui*), uncooked Radix Astragali Membranacei (*Huang Qi*)

5. *Si Wu Tang Jia Pao Jiang:* Prepared Radix Rehmanniae (*Shu Di*), Radix Albus Paeoniae Lactiflorae (*Bai Shao*), Radix Angelicae Sinensis (*Dang Gui*), Radix Ligustici Wallichii (*Chuan Xiong*), blast-fried Rhizoma Zingiberis (*Pao Jiang*)

171

6. *Si Wu Tang Jia Pao Jiang Shen Shu:* Prepared Radix Rehmanniae (*Shu Di*), Radix Albus Paeoniae Lactiflorae (*Bai Shao*), Radix Angelicae Sinensis (*Dang Gui*), Radix Ligustici Wallichii (*Chuan Xiong*), blast-fried Rhizoma Zingiberis (*Pao Jiang*), Radix Panacis Ginseng (*Ren Shen*), Rhizoma Atractylodis Macrocephalae (*Bai Zhu*)

7. *Sheng Yu Tang:* See Section Six, Chapter Four.

Section Three

Postpartum Lochia Does Not Cease (*Chan Hou E Lu Bu Jue*)

If the postpartum lochia continues for more than 3 weeks, dribbling and dripping without cease, this is called lochia which does not cease (*e lu bu jue*) or lochia which is not complete (*e lou bu jing*). If the lochia continues for many days and is not stopped, this commonly results in fluid exhaustion. This easily engenders other diseases and thus should be promptly treated.

Disease Causes, Disease Mechanisms

The causes of the onset of this disease are typically divided into three types: 1) Vacuity detriment of the *chong* and *ren* which are not able to secure and contain. If postpartum the discharge of blood is excessive, this may damage the *chong* and *ren* resulting in qi and blood becoming irregular. Thus the lochia does not cease. 2) Static blood may not stay within limits. It ceases and is retained in the uterus. Thus the blood cannot return to the channels. 3) Liver channel blood heat may force the blood to move recklessly.

Disease Patterns

Chong & Ren Not Securing

The lochia does not cease. The color of the blood is pale and yellowish. The facial complexion is somber white or sallow yellow. There is essence spirit fatigue, bodily emaciation and weakness, fear of chill, dizziness, vertigo, heart palpitations, tinnitus, chest oppression, shortness of breath, a soft abdominal region, abdominal pain which likes pressure, a pale red tongue with scanty coating, and a vacuous, fine, weak pulse.

Static Blood Not Within Limits

The postpartum lochia does not stop. There may be blood clots which are purple in color. There is a foul odor or it is filthy and turbid. There is lower abdominal aching and pain, a purple, dark tongue, and a wiry, choppy pulse.

Liver Channel Blood Heat

The postpartum lochia does nor cease. There is heat vexation, dry mouth, a red tongue, and a fine, rapid or wiry, rapid pulse.

Treatment

Chong & Ren Not Securing

One should warm and nourish, secure and contain. The formula to use is *Shi Quan Da Bu Tang* (Ten [Ingredients] Greatly & Completely Supplementing Decoction). This supplements the qi and nourishes the blood. In order to restrain, astringe, and secure desertion, the formula to use is *Mu Li San* (Oyster Shell Powder). For qi vacuity and downward falling, the formula to use is *Qian Jin Sheng Ma Tang* (*Thousand [Pieces of] Gold* Cimicifuga Decoction). For blood vacuity abdominal pain, the formula to use is *Jia Wei Si Wu Tang* (Added Flavors Four Materials Decoction). And

173

for postpartum excessive discharge of blood with qi vacuity not able to gather the blood, use *Si Wu Tang* (Four Materials Decoction) plus Gelatinum Corii Asini (*E Jiao*), Radix Panacis Ginseng (*Ren Shen*), Radix Astragali Membranacei (*Huang Qi*), and Terra Flava Usta (*Fu Long Gan*).

Static Blood Not Within Limits

One should quicken the blood and dispel stasis. The formula to use is *Sheng Hua Tang* (Engendering & Transforming Decoction) or *Shi Xiao San* (Sudden Smile Powder). If there is bodily vacuity and chilled limbs, add Cortex Cinnamomi (*Rou Gui*). If heat is heavy, remove Cortex Cinnamomi (*Rou Gui*) and blast-fried Rhizoma Zingiberis (*Pao Jiang*) and add Fructus Gardeniae Jasminoidis (*Shan Zhi*), Cortex Radicis Moutan (*Dan Pi*), and wine stir-fried Radix Scutellariae Baicalensis (*Huang Qin*). If there is abdominal pain, add Radix Linderae Strychnifoliae (*Wu Yao*), Fructus Meliae Toosendan (*Chuan Lian Zi*), and Rhizoma Corydalis Yanhusuo (*Yan Hu Suo*). For excessive discharge of blood, add Radix Panacis Ginseng (*Ren Shen*), Radix Astragali Membranacei (*Huang Qi*), and carbonized Petiolus Trachycarpi (*Zong Lu Tan*).

Liver Channel Blood Heat

One should nourish yin and clear heat. The formula to use is *Pao Yin Jian* (Protect Yin Decoction), *Qing Hua Yin* (Clear & Transform Drink), or something of that type.

Explanation

For the effective treatment of postpartum lochia which does not cease, one should discriminate vacuity and repletion since these are not the same patterns. For qi and blood dual deficiency, supplement the qi and nourish the blood. For static blood internally obstructing, dispel stasis and engender the new. For liver channel blood heat, one should clear heat and nourish the blood. If there chances to be cold, warm the channels and gather the blood. If simultaneously there is aversion to cold and fever due to common cold, treatment should course and resolve, diffuse and reach. If there is liver qi depression and binding with chest fullness and counterflow qi, treatment should course the liver and resolve depression. If internally food is stopped and lodged, one should disperse food and abduct stagnation at the same time as supporting the spleen.

Appended Formulas

1. *Shi Quan Da Bu Tang:* See Section Six, Chapter Four.

2. *Mu Li San (*from *Zheng Zhi Zhun Sheng [Proven Treatments Norms & Restrictions]):* Calcined Concha Ostreae (*Mu Li*), Radix Ligustici Wallichii (*Chuan Xiong*), prepared Radix Rehmanniae (*Shu Di*), Sclerotium Poriae Cocos (*Fu Ling*), Os Draconis (*Long Gu*), Radix Dipsaci (*Xu Duang*), wine stir-fried Radix Angelicae Sinensis (*Dang Gui*), stir-fried Folium Artemisiae Argyii (*Ai Ye*), Radix Panacis Ginseng (*Ren Shen*), Fructus Schizandrae Chinensis (*Wu Wei Zi*), carbonized Radix Sanguisorbae (*Di Yu*), Radix Glycyrrhizae (*Gan Cao*), uncooked Rhizoma Zingiberis (*Sheng Jiang*), Fructus Zizyphi Jujubae (*Da Zao*)

3. *Qian Jin Sheng Ma Tang (*from *Qian Jin Yao Fang [Formulas {Worth a} Thousand {Pieces of} Gold]):* Green Rhizoma Cimicifugae (*Sheng Ma*). Decoct with wine and take warm.

4. *Jia Wei Si Wu Tang:* Prepared Radix Rehmanniae (*Shu Di*), Radix Albus Paeoniae Lactiflorae (*Bai Shao*), Radix Angelicae Sinensis (*Dang Gui*), Radix Ligustici Wallichii (*Chuan Xiong*), Gelatinum Corii Asini (*E Jiao*), Radix Panacis Ginseng (*Ren Shen*), Radix Astragali Membranacei (*Huang Qi*), Terra Flava Usta (*Fu Long Gan*)

5. *Sheng Hua Tang:* See Section Five, Chapter Six.

6. *Shi Xiao San:* See Section Ten, Chapter Four.

7. *Bao Yin Jian:* See Section Two, Chapter Five.

8. *Qing Hua Yin* (from *Jing Yue Quan Shu [Jing-yue's Complete Writings])*: Radix Albus Paeoniae Lactiflorae (*Bai Shao*), Tuber Ophiopogonis Japonicae (*Mai Dong*), Sclerotium Poriae Cocos (*Fu Ling*), Radix Scutellariae Baicalensis (*Huang Qin*), uncooked Radix Rehmanniae (*Sheng Di*), Herba Dendrobii (*Shi Hu*)

Section Four

Postpartum Blood Dizziness (*Chan Hou Xue Yun*)

Postpartum blood dizziness is called depressed stomach (*yu wei*) in the *Jin Gui Yao Lue (Essentials from the Golden Cabinet)*. This refers to women who, after parturition, have dizziness, vertigo, black flowers in front of the eyes, dimness and oppression on the verge of cessation (*i.e.*, faintness), and loss of consciousness of human affairs. If severe, there is aphasia, no speech, and other such symptoms. This is called postpartum blood dizziness.

Disease Causes, Disease Mechanisms

The cause of the onset of this disease is mainly excessive expulsion of blood in the newly birthed. the blood is vacuous and thus there is inversion. The *Jin Gui Yao Lue (Essentials from the Golden Cabinet)* says:

> Because of blood vacuity, there is inversion; because of inversion, there is faintness.

This points out that there is blood vacuity and qi inversion counterflowing upward. Thus there are the symptoms of dimness, dizziness, desperation, and oppression. Xue Li-zhai also says:

> Postpartum the original qi is deficient and has suffered detriment. Thus the lochia takes advantage of vacuity and attacks upward.

The *Fu Ren Da Quan Liang Fang (A Great, Complete [Collection] of Fine Formulas for Women)* says:

> Postpartum blood dizziness is due to vanquished blood flowing into the liver channel. Thus the eyes are dim and dark. One cannot see things clearly and one cannot rise from sitting.

As suggested by the above quotations, the causes of postpartum blood dizziness are none other than blood vacuity, qi vacuity, and blood stasis, these three types.

Disease Patterns

Blood Vacuity

After delivery, the birthing woman has expelled excessive blood. There is dizziness, vertigo, blurred, confused vision, and inability to rise from sitting. If severe, there is oppression and desperation, loss of consciousness of human affairs, aphasia, speechlessness, a white facial complexion and somber white lips. There is sweat on the forehead, a pale tongue, and a minute, weak pulse.

Qi Vacuity

The symptoms are similar to those of blood vacuity. However, the birthing woman during pregnancy was bodily emaciated and weak, and qi and blood were insufficient. After parturition, the essence spirit is fatigued and there occur clouding, oppression, and loss of consciousness of human affairs. The face is a somber white, the four limbs have inversion chill, the mouth is chilled or there is phlegm congestion. There is excessive sweating from the forehead, the tongue is pale with a thin coating, and the pulse is vacuous, fine, and forceless.

177

Blood Stasis

The symptoms are similar to those of blood vacuity. However, the lochia is scanty, the face and lips are red in color or purple and dark. There is lower abdominal distention and pain which refuses pressure. The tongue is purple and dark, and the pulse is deep and stagnant.

Treatment

No matter whether the patient is vacuous or replete, whenever there is blood dizziness and lack of knowledge of human affairs, have the patient inhale the steam produced by dipping a heated iron into vinegar. Or one can pierce the center of the eyebrows (*i.e.*, *Yin Tang* [M-HN-3]) and exit blood at the same time as moxaing the two points *Bai Hui* (GV 20) and *Guan Yuan* (CV 4). After these symptoms are relieved, administer internal medicinal treatment.

Blood Vacuity

After using the above emergency methods, supplement by using a large dose of *Xiong Gui Tang* (Ligusticum & Dang Gui Decoction), decocted in water and administered at no set time. If there is abdominal pain, add wine stir-fried Radix Albus Paeoniae Lactiflorae (*Bai Shao*) and Cortex Cinnamomi (*Rou Gui*). If there is a dry mouth and vexatious thirst, add Fructus Pruni Mume (*Wu Mei*) and Tuber Ophiopogonis Japonicae (*Mai Dong*). If there is emission of cold and heat, add dry Rhizoma Zingiberis (*Gan Jiang*) and Radix Albus Paeoniae Lactiflorae (*Bai Shao*). If water ceases below the heart and there is slight nausea, add Sclerotium Poriae Cocos (*Fu Ling*) and uncooked Rhizoma Zingiberis (*Sheng Jiang*). And if there is vacuity vexation and no sleep, add Radix Panacis Ginseng (*Ren Shen*) and Folium Bambusae (*Zhu Ye*).

Qi Vacuity

One should supplement the qi and boost the blood. The formula to use is *Bu Qi Jie Yun Tang* (Supplement the Qi & Resolve Dizziness Decoction) or *Qing Hun San* (Clear the Ethereal Soul Powder). If qi and blood are both empty, one can use *Shi Quan Da Bu Tang* (Ten [Ingredients] Greatly & Completely Supplementing Decoction).

Blood Stasis

One should mainly dispel stasis. The formula to use is *Shi Xiao San* (Sudden Smile Powder), *Duo Ming San* (Seize One's Destiny Powder). If there is simultaneous wind evils accompanied by cold and heat, headache, a bluish tongue with a thin, white coating, and a floating, astringent pulse, one can use *Jing Jie San* (Schizonepeta Powder). If there is slight panting, add Semen Pruni Armeniacae (*Xing Ren*) and stir-fried Radix Glycyrrhizae (*Gan Cao*). If accompanied by cold evils, *i.e.*, the previous symptoms and a bluish, ashen facial complexion, chilled limbs and abdomen, loose stools, and a deep, tight, choppy pulse, one should mainly use *Hei Shen San* (Black Spirit Powder). If accompanied by qi depression, *i.e.*, the previous symptoms and a somber, dark facial complexion, chest and epigastric fullness and oppression, abdominal distention and pain, a bluish, dark tongue with a thin, sticky coating, and a wiry, choppy pulse, one should mainly use *Yu Jin San Jia Wei* (Jade & Gold Powder with Added Flavors). If the previous symptoms are accompanied by heat, a red face and lips, confusion and chaos, internal heat, a dry mouth, constipation, a red tongue with a thin, yellow coating, and a rapid pulse, one should mainly use *Tong Yu Yin* (Open Stasis Drink) or *Hong Hua San* (Carthamus Powder).

Explanation

1. Postpartum blood dizziness is mostly caused by constitutional vacuity weakness, prolonged labor, and overuse of force during delivery.

2. In the treatment of postpartum blood dizziness, if one has only used medicinals which move stasis and has not gotten good results, one can add moving qi medicinals, such as carbonized Rhizoma Cyperi Rotundi (*Xiang Fu*) and carbonized Radix Linderae Strychnifoliae (*Wu Yao*). This will improve the results.

3. If the patient is perplexed by frequent attacks of faintness accompanied by numbness of the whole body and cold limbs which do not show any sign of improvement even after drinking decoctions containing Radix Panacis Ginseng (*Ren Shen*) and Radix Astragali Membranacei (*Huang Qi*), this is due to static blood obstructing and stagnating. The transportation of blood is not smoothly flowing. One can use quickening the blood and moving stasis medicinals, such as Resina Myrrhae (*Mo Yao*) and Sanguis Draconis (*Xue Jie*), 3g each, mixed with yellow (*i.e.*, rice) wine (*Huang Jiu*) and taken. This usually gets a good result.

4. In order to prevent dimness and dizziness, one can take a mixture made of inkstick and vinegar. Heat the inkstick until it becomes glowing red. Dip into a jar of vinegar. Repeat this process 7 times. Then grind the inkstick into fine powder for use. The usual dosage is 3-6g taken with dilute vinegar soup or wine immediately after delivery.

Appended Formulas

1. *Xiong Gui Tang:* See Section Three, Chapter Six.

2. *Bu Qi Jie Yun Tang (*from *Fu Qing Zhu Nu Ke [Fu Qing-zhu's Gynecology]):* Radix Panacis Ginseng (*Ren Shen*), uncooked Radix Astragali Membranacei (*Huang Qi*), Radix Angelicae Sinensis (*Dang Gui*), blackened Herba Seu Flos Schizonepetae Tenuifoliae (*Jing Jie*), carbonized Rhizoma Zingiberis (*Jiang*)

3. *Qing Hun San (*from *Ji Sheng Fang [Formulas for the Aid of the Living]):* Folium Lycopi Lucidi (*Ze Lan Ye*), Radix Panacis Ginseng (*Ren Shen*), Radix Ligustici Wallichii (*Chuan Xiong*), Herba Seu Flos Schizonepetae Tenuifoliae (*Jing Jie*), Radix Glycyrrhizae (*Gan Cao*)

4. *Shi Quan Da Bu Tang:* See Section Five, Chapter Four.

5. *Shi Xiao San:* See Section Ten, Chapter, Four.

6. *Duo Ming San (*from *Ji Yin Gang Mu [Detailed Outline of Yin]): */ Resina Myrrhae (*Mo Yao*), Sanguis Draconis (*Xue Jie*). Grind equal parts into fine powder and take with infant's urine and wine.

7. *Jing Jie San (*from *Ji Yin Gang Mu [Detailed Outline of Yin]):* Herba Seu Flos Schizonepetae Tenuifoliae (*Jing Jie*), Semen Pruni Persicae (*Tao Ren*). Grind into powder and take 9g each time with warm wine.

8. *Hei Shen San (*from *Tai Ping Hui Min He Ji Ju Fang [Tai Ping Imperial Grace Formulary]):* Radix Angelicae Sinensis (*Dang Gui*), Radix Albus Paeoniae Lactiflorae (*Bai Shao*), prepared Radix Rehmanniae (*Shu Di Huang*), blast-fried dry Rhizoma Zingiberis (*Pao Gan Jiang*), Cortex Cinnamomi (*Rou Gui*), Pollen Typhae (*Pu Huang*), mix-fried Radix Glycyrrhizae (*Zhi Gan Cao*), stir-fried, skin-removed Semen Glycinis Hispidae (*Hei Dou*), 1/2 *jin*. Grind the above into fine powder and take 9g each time, with 1/2 teacup each of infant's urine and wine.

9. *Yu Jing San (*from *Yi Lue Liu Shu [A Synopsis of Medicine in Six Books]):* Grind the residue of Szechuan Tuber Curcumae (*Yu Jin*) into powder and take 9g each time, mixed with infant's urine and vinegar.

10. *Tong Yu Yin Jia Wei (*from *Shen Shi Zun Sheng Shu [Master Shen's Writings on Respecting Life]):* Radix Angelicae Sinensis tails (*Gui Wei*), Radix Et Rhizoma Rhei (*Da Huang*), Rhizoma Atractylodis Macrocephalae (*Bai Zhu*), Caulis Akebiae Mutong (*Mu Tong*), Flos Carthami Tinctorii (*Hong Hua*), Semen Pruni Persicae (*Tao Ren*), Cortex Radicis Moutan (*Dan Pi*), Pollen Typhae (*Pu Huang*), Radix Achyranthis Bidentatae (*Niu Xi*)

11. *Hong Hua San (*from *Pao Ming Fang [Destiny-protecting Formulas]):* Dry Folium Nelumbinis Nuciferae (*He Ye*), Cortex Radicis Moutan (*Dan Pi*), Radix Angelicae Sinensis (*Dang Gui*), Flos Carthami Tinctorii (*Hong Hua*), stir-fried Pollen Typhae (*Pu Huang*)

181

Section Five

Postpartum Fever (*Chan Hou Fa Re*)

If a birthing woman after parturition has a continuous fever which does not resolve associated with other symptoms, this is called postpartum fever, *chan hou fa re*.

Disease Causes, Disease Mechanisms

Postpartum fever has many causes. For example, excessive eating and drinking may cause vomiting and aversion to food. This may cause food damage fever. If one gets up too early and overtaxes themself, they may be invaded by wind cold. This leads to external invasion fever. If the lochia is not discharged, static blood may cease and be retained. This may lead to static blood fever. If the expelled blood is too much, yin blood may become insufficient. This leads to blood vacuity fever. It may also be caused by taxation and overexertion during birthing resulting in fever, or 3 days of steaming milk (*i.e.*, mastitis) resulting in fever. In addition, due to lack of care during delivery, there may be inadvertent damage and detriment to the birth canal, or there may be improper nursing of the external genitalia, resulting in invasion of toxic evils and thus fever.

Disease Patterns

External Invasion Fever

There is aversion to cold, fever, a sallow yellow facial complexion, bodily emaciation, essence spirit fatigue, headache, dizziness, low back soreness, bone pain, possible qi panting and cough, possible head and neck pulling pain, or nausea and vomiting. The tongue is pale red with a thin, white coating. The pulse is floating and fine.

Food Damage Fever

There is chest and diaphragmatic satiation and oppression, hiccup, acid eructation, no thought for food or drink, discomfort caused by eating, epigastric and abdominal distention and pain, possible vomiting and diarrhea, a filthy, slimy tongue coating, and a slippery, rapid pulse.

Static Blood Fever

There is lower abdominal distention, fullness, and pain aggravated by pressure, a scanty lochia or discharge of a small amount of purple, dark static clots, a dark, purplish tongue, and a wiry, choppy pulse.

Blood Vacuity Fever

Postpartum the qi and blood are already deficient, yin is vacuous and yang floats. Qi and blood are both vacuous, and there is tinnitus, heart palpitations, scanty sleep, and possible constipation. Or premature overtaxation may cause bodily vacuity resulting in fever and fear of chill. There is tidal fever or cold and heat coming alternately. The facial complexion is a somber white and there is dizziness, vertigo, essence spirit fatigue, low back and knee soreness and weakness, a pale tongue without coating, and a fine, minute pulse.

Steaming Milk Fever

Two to three days after birthing, there is aversion to cold, fever, breast distention and pain, hard lumps revealed by pressure, and inability of the breast milk to flow freely. The tongue is pale red, and the pulse is wiry and rapid.

Invasion by Toxic Evils Fever

There is fever, aversion to cold, or alternating cold and heat, perspiration, lower abdominal pain which refuses pressure, either an excessive or scanty lochia which is purplish black in color and smells bad, vexation and agitation, oral thirst, a red face, constipation, and short, reddish urination. If severe, there is high fever which does not recede, spirit clouding, delirious speech, and macules and rashes appearing on the skin. The tongue is red with a yellow coating or scarlet with a thick, yellow, dry coating. The pulse is surging and rapid or wiry, fine, and rapid.

Treatment

External Invasion Fever

One should resolve the exterior and simultaneously nourish the blood. The formula to use is *Zhu Ye Tang* (Bamboo Leaf Decoction) or *Zeng Sun Chai Hu Tang* (Augment Detriment Bupleurum Decoction).

Food Damage Fever

One should disperse food and fortify the spleen. The formula to use is *Jia Wei Si Jun Zi Tang* (Added Flavors Four Gentlemen Decoction).

Static Blood Fever

One should move the blood and dispel stasis. The formula to use is *Sheng Hua Tang* (Engendering & Transforming Decoction), *Shi Xiao San* (Sudden Smile Powder).

Blood Vacuity Fever

One should greatly supplement the qi and blood. The formula to use is *Shi Quan Da Bu Tang* (Ten [Ingredients] Greatly & Completely Supplementing Decoction) or *Ren Shen Dang Gui Tang* (Ginseng & Dang Gui Decoction). If there is alternating cold and heat, one can use *Xiao Chai Hu Tang* (Minor Bupleurum Decoction) plus *Sheng Di Huang Tang* (Uncooked Rehmannia Decoction). If there is postpartum many days enduring vacuity taxation fever, one can use *San He San* (Three Unitings Powder).

Steaming Milk Fever

One should smooth and free the flow of milk and then cold and heat will automatically recede. The formula to use is *Gua Lou San* (Trichosanthes Powder), the dregs of which can be decocted again with which to warm and wash the breast. Or one may drink a soup made from 60g of Fructus Germinatus Hordei Vulgaris (*Mai Ya*) in order to return the milk (*i.e.,* stop lactation).

Invasion by Toxic Evils Fever

One should clear heat and resolve toxins, quicken the blood and transform stasis. The formula to use is *Qing Re Jie Du Tang* (Clear Heat & Resolve Toxins Decoction). Radix Scutellariae Baicalensis (*Huang Qin*) and Radix Bupleuri (*Chai Hu*) can be added if accompanied by alternating cold and heat. If there is high fever which does not recede, oral thirst leading to drinking, rough breathing, excessive sweating, and a surging, large pulse, this is categorized as heat toxins internally harassing the lungs and stomach. One should clear and drain heat from the lungs and stomach. The formula to use is *Ren Shen Bai Hu Tang* (Ginseng White Tiger Decoction) plus Flos Lonicerae Japonicae (*Jin Yin Hua*) and Fructus Forsythiae Suspensae (*Lian Qiao*). However, if there is severe lower abdominal pain, unsmooth flow of the lochia, constipation, and a high fever which does not recede, use *Da Huang Mu Dan Pi Tang* (Rhubarb & Moutan Decoction). If heat enters the constructive and blood, the commonly seen pattern is high fever, spirit clouding, delirious speech, and macules and rashes appearing on the skin. One can use *An Gong Niu Huang Wan* (Quiet the Palace Bezoar Pills) or *Zhi Xue Dan* (Purple Snow Elixir).

Explanation

Although postpartum fever may manifest various patterns, really there is nothing other than internal damage fever and external invasion fever, these two types. In terms of diagnosis, carefully analyzing the pulse image for whether it is floating and rapid or deep and rapid and intensively observing the tongue coating as to whether it is slimy or glossy are of utmost importance. In addition, sweating or no sweating and exterior heat or interior heat should each be distinguished one from the other. If there is heat in the exterior pattern, one should first resolve the exterior. However, when resolving the exterior, one should take into account blood vacuity. Therefore, it is said, "Speed the soldiers' assault, especially if lacking a rear guard." Once there is sweating, there is resolution. One should not overuse acrid, scattering medicinals. If sometimes there is chill and sometimes there is fever, the disease is located in the *shao yang*. Therefore one can use *Xiao Chai Hu Tang Jia Jian* (Minor Bupleurum Decoction with Additions & Subtractions). One or two heavy doses are able to cure. If high fever appears with oral thirst, great sweating, a surging, and large pulse, in order to clear the qi and recede heat, the formula to use is *Ren Shen Bai Hu Tang Jia Jian* (Ginseng White Tiger Decoction with Additions & Subtractions). If evils have entered the constructive and blood and there is high fever which does not recede, spirit clouding, and delirious speech, in order to assist the clearing of heat and resolution of toxins described above, add *An Gong Niu Huang Wan* (Quiet the Palace Bezoar Pills) or *Zhi Xue Dan* (Purple Snow Elixir) to clear heat and open the portals, thus rescuing an emergency.

Appended Formulas

1. *Zhu Ye Tang (*from *Jin Gui Yao Lue [Essentials from the Golden Cabinet]):* Folium Bambusae (*Zhu Ye*), Radix Ledebouriellae Sesloidis (*Fang Feng*), Radix Puerariae (*Ge Gen*), Radix Platycodi Grandiflori (*Jie Geng*, Ramulus Cinnamomi (*Gui Zhi*), Radix Panacis Ginseng (*Ren Shen*), mix-fried Radix Glycyrrhizae (*Zhi Gan Cao*), Radix Lateralis Praeparatus Aconiti Carmichaeli (*Shu Fu Zi*), Fructus Zizyphi Jujubae (*Da Zao*), uncooked Rhizoma Zingiberis (*Sheng Jiang*)

2. *Zeng Sun Chai Hu Tang (*from *Zheng Zhi Zhun Sheng [Patterns & Treatments Norms & Criteria]):* Radix Bupleuri (*Chai Hu*), Radix Panacis Ginseng (*Ren Shen*), Radix Glycyrrhizae (*Gan Cao*), processed Rhizoma Pinelliae Ternatae (*Ban Xia*), Pericarpium Citri Reticulatae (*Chen Pi*), Radix Ligustici Wallichii (*Chuan Xiong*), Radix Albus Paeoniae Lacti-

florae (*Bai Shao*), uncooked Rhizoma Zingiberis (*Sheng Jiang*), Fructus Zizyphi Jujubae (*Da Zao*)

3. *Jia Wei Si Jun Zi Tang:* Radix Panacis Ginseng (*Ren Shen*), Rhizoma Praeparata Atractylodis Macrocephalae, Sclerotium Poriae Cocos (*Fu Ling*), mix-fried Radix Glycyrrhizae (Zhi Gan Cao), Rhizoma Praeparata Pinelliae, Pericarpium Citri Reticulatae, Fructus Seu Semen Amomi, Massa Medica Fermentata, uncooked Rhizoma Zingiberis (*Sheng Jiang*), and Fructus Zizyphi Jujubae (*Da Zao*).

4. *Sheng Hua Tang:* See Section Five, Chapter Six.

5. *Shi Xiao San:* See Section Ten, Chapter Four.

6. *Shi Quan Da Bu Tang:* See Section Five, Chapter Four.

7. *Ren Shen Dang Gui Tang (*from *Zheng Zhi Zhun Sheng [Patterns & Treatments Norms & Criteria]):* Radix Panacis Ginseng (*Ren Shen*), Radix Angelicae Sinensis (*Dang Gui*), prepared Radix Rehmanniae (*Shu Di*), Cortex Cinnamomi (*Rou Gui*), Tuber Ophiopogonis Japonicae (*Mai Dong*), Radix Albus Paeoniae Lactiflorae (*Bai Shao*), Herba Lophatheri Gracilis (*Dan Zhu Ye*), Fructus Oryzae Sativae (*Geng Mi*), Fructus Zizyphi Jujubae (*Da Zao*)

8. *Xiao Chai Hu Tang* plus *Sheng Di Huang Tang:* Radix Bupleuri (*Chai Hu*), Radix Scutellariae Baicalensis (*Huang Qin*), Fructus Gardeniae Jasminoidis (*Shan Zhi*), Radix Panacis Ginseng (*Ren Shen*), uncooked Radix Rehmanniae (*Sheng Di*), Fructus Citri Seu Ponciri (*Zhi Ke*), Rhizoma Pinelliae Ternatae (*Ban Xia*)

9. *San He San (*from *Zheng Zhi Zhun Sheng [Patterns & Treatments Norms & Criteria]):* Radix Ligustici Wallichii (*Chuan Xiong*), Radix Angelicae Sinensis (*Dang Gui*), stir-fried Radix Albus Paeoniae Lactiflorae (*Bai Shao*), prepared Radix Rehmanniae (*Shu Di*), stir-fried Rhizoma Atractylodis Macrocephalae (*Bai Zhu*), Sclerotium Poriae Cocos (*Fu Ling*), mix-fried Radix Astragali Membranacei (*Huang Qi*), Radix Bupleuri (*Chai Hu*),

187

Radix Panacis Ginseng (*Ren Shen*), Radix Scutellariae Baicalensis (*Huang Qin*), processed Rhizoma Pinelliae Ternatae (*Ban Xia*), mix-fried Radix Glycyrrhizae (*Zhi Gan Cao*), uncooked Rhizoma Zingiberis (*Sheng Jiang*), Fructus Zizyphi Jujubae (*Da Zao*)

10. *Gua Lou San (*from *Ji Yin Gang Mu [Detailed Outline of Yin]):* Stir-fried Fructus Trichosanthis Kirlowii (*Gua Lou*), Radix Glycyrrhizae (*Gan Cao*), blast-fried Rhizoma Zingiberis (*Pao Jiang*). Decoct in 2 bowls of wine and take.

11. *Qing Re Jie Du Tang* (an empirical formula): Flos Lonicerae Japonicae (*Jin Yin Hua*), Fructus Forsythiae (*Lian Qiao*), Herba Cum Radice Taraxaci Mongolici (*Pu Gong Ying*), Herba Violae Yedoensis (*Zi Di Ding*), Cortex Radicis Moutan (*Dan Pi*), Herba Leonuri Heterophylli (*Yi Mu Cao*), Radix Albus Paeoniae Lactiflorae (*Bai Shao*), Pollen Typhae (*Pu Huang*)

12. *Ren Shen Bai Hu Tang (*from *Shang Han Lun [Treatise on Damage Due to Cold]):* Gypsum Fibrosum (*Shi Gao*), Radix Panacis Ginseng (*Ren Shen*), Fructus Oryzae Sativae (*Geng Mi*), Rhizoma Anemarrhenae (*Zhi Mu*), Radix Glycyrrhizae (*Gan Cao*)

13. *Da Huang Mu Dan Pi Tang (*from *Jin Gui Yao Lue [Essentials from the Golden Cabinet]):* Semen Pruni Persicae (*Tao Ren*), Mirabilitum (*Mang Xiao*), Cortex Radicis Moutan (*Dan Pi*), Radix Et Rhizoma Rhei (*Da Huang*), Semen Benincasae Hispidae (*Dong Gua Zi*)

14. *An Gong Niu Huang Wan (*from *Wen Bing Tiao Bian [The Discrimination of Warm Diseases]):* Calculus Bovis (*Niu Huang*), Tuber Curcumae (*Yu Jin*), Cornu Rhinocerotis (*Xi Jiao*, substitute Cornu Bubali [*Shui Niu Jiao*]), Radix Scutellariae Baicalensis, Rhizoma Coptidis Chinensis (*Huang Lian*), Realgar (*Xiong Huang*), Fructus Gardeniae Jasminoidis (*Zhi Zi*), Cinnabar (*Zhu Sha*), Borneol (*Mu Pian)*, Secretio Moschi Moschiferi (*She Xiang*), Margarita (*Zhen Mu*)

15. *Zhi Xue Dan (*from *Wen Bing Tiao Bian [The Discrimination of Warm Diseases]):* Talcum (*Hua Shi*), Gypsum Fibrosum (*Shi Gao*), Calcitum

(*Han Shui Shi*), Magnetitum (*Ci Shi*), Cornu Antelopis (*Ling Yang Jiao*), Radix Saussureae Seu Vladimiriae (*Mu Xiang*), Cornu Rhinocerotis (*Xi Jiao*, substitute Cornu Bubali [*Shui Niu Jiao*]), Lignum Aquilariae Agallochae (*Chen Xiang*), Flos Caryophylli (*Ding Xiang*), Rhizoma Cimicifugae (*Sheng Ma*), Radix Scrophulariae Ningpoensis (*Xuan Shen*), mix-fried Radix Glycyrrhizae (*Zhi Gan Cao*), Mirabilitum (*Mang Xiao*), Cinnabar (*Zhu Sha*), Secretio Moschi Moschiferi (*She Xiang*)

Section Six

Postpartum Tetany (*Chan Hou Fa Jing*)

Sudden convulsive seizures and neck and upper back rigidity, tremors and contracture of the four limbs, if severe, lockjaw, and opisthotonos occurring after childbirth are called *chan hou fa jing* or postpartum tetany.

Disease Causes, Disease Mechanisms

The cause of postpartum tetany is mainly due to excessive expulsion of blood during parturition. It may also be due to excessive force being used during birthing with excessive perspiration. The constructive and blood are greatly deficient and this results in liver channel blood vacuity. The sinew vessels thus lose their moisture and liver wind is engendered internally. If sweating is excessive, the skin is empty and open and the interstices are not densely packed. Wind evils may take advantage of vacuity and enter, causing the teeth to be tightly closed, the neck to be rigid and arched, opisthotonos, and other such symptoms. As it is said in the Yi Zong Jin Jian (Golden Mirror of Ancestral Medicine):

> Postpartum blood and qi are insufficient, the viscera and bowels are all vacuous. If there is excessive discharge of sweat, the interstices are not densely packed. Wind evils take advantage of vacuity and invade, thus producing tetany disease.

Xue Li-zhai has also said:

> Postpartum tetany is due to excessive expulsion of blood, original qi
> deficiency, or external evils mutually wrestling.

Thus this disease's disease causes are mostly blood vacuity leading to the
arising of internal wind and external wind invasion, these two types.

Disease Patterns

Blood Vacuity

During parturition excessive blood is expelled. There is a stiff, arched neck,
opisthotonos, lockjaw and aphasia, tremors and contracture of the four
limbs, both hands tightly shut, possible inversion counterflow of the hands
and feet, twitching of the mouth and eyes, pale white colored lips and face,
and a wiry, fine or floating, scattered, forceless pulse image.

Wind Cold

After parturition, there is fear of cold, fever, headache, soreness and pain
of the bones and joints, sudden lockjaw, aphasia, upward staring eyes,
possible opisthotonos, tremors and contracture of the hands and feet, and
a floating, wiry pulse.

Treatment

Blood Vacuity

One should nourish the blood and extinguish wind. The formula to use is
Ba Zhen Tang (Eight Pearls Decoction) plus Cortex Radicis Moutan (*Dan
Pi*), Ramulus Uncariae Cum Uncis (*Gou Teng*), and uncooked Radix
Rehmanniae (*Sheng Di*). If there is inversion of the four limbs, a somber
white facial complexion, a floating, scattered pulse, and no spirit, for

190

emergency use *Shi Quan Da Bu Tang* (Ten [Ingredients] Greatly & Completely Supplementing Decoction) plus Radix Lateralis Praeparatus Aconiti Carmichaeli (*Fu Zi*) to salvage. If the sinew vessels are not constructed and there are contracture and spasms of the four limbs, one can use *Zi Rong Huo Xue Tang* (Enrich the Constructive & Quicken the Blood Decoction). And for blood vacuity with vanquished blood surging into the heart, *Qi Zhen San* (Seven Pearls Powder) is the treatment.

Wind Cold

One should nourish the blood and course wind, assisted by quickening the blood and resolving the exterior. If the birthing woman fears chill and has fever, headache, soreness and pain of the bones and joints, lockjaw which does not open, opisthotonos, and contracture and spasm of the four limbs, *Yu Feng Tang* (Healing Wind Decoction), *Dang Gui San* (Dang Gui Powder) and *Tian Ma San* (Gastrodia Powder) treat this.

Explanation

1. In the *Yi Zong Jin Jian (Golden Mirror of Ancestral Medicine)*, the treatment of postpartum tetany is divided into wind stroke, clonic convulsions, contracture and spasms, and aphasia, these four types. In general, these are the result of postpartum perishing of blood damaging fluids and excessive sweating resulting in blood vacuity with the sinew vessels not being constructed. Thus there is blood vacuity and stirring of wind. The *Jin Gui Yao Lue (Essentials from the Golden Cabinet]* also points out:

> In the newly birthed, blood vacuity and excessive sweating causes susceptibility to wind stroke and thus the production of tetany disease.

In addition, the *Yi Zong Jin Jian (Golden Mirror of Ancestral Medicine)* has it that first one should mainly greatly supplement the qi and blood. Other symptoms are taken as secondary aspects and can be treated after the signs of this disease have mostly been eliminated.

191

2. If the newly birthed woman has expelled excessive blood, she must have a timid heart and feel weak. Therefore, it is very important to protect the patient from noise lest convulsions manifest due to fright.

3. If due to heat phlegm misting the heart, one can administer *Shen Shi Nu Ke Dan Xing Xuan Qiao Fang* (*Master Shen's Gynecology* Bile(-processed) Arisaema Diffuse the Portals Formula): bile(-processed) Rhizoma Arisaematis (*Dan Xing*), Exocarpium Citri Erythrocarpae (*Ju Hong*), ginger(-processed) Rhizoma Pinelliae Ternatae (*Ban Xia*), Rhizoma Acori Graminei (*Shi Chang Pu*), Tuber Curcumae (*Yu Jin*), Succus Bambusae (Zhu Li), and the juice from uncooked Rhizoma Zingiberis (*Sheng Jiang*).

Appended Formulas

1. *Ba Zhen Tang:* See Section Two, Chapter Five.

2. *Shi Quan Da Bu Tang:* See Section Five, Chapter Four.

3. *Zi Rong Huo Xue Tang* (from *Fu Qing Zhu Nu Ke [Fu Qing-zhu's Gynecology]*): Radix Ligustici Wallichii (*Chuan Xiong*), Radix Angelicae Sinensis (*Dang Gui*), prepared Radix Rehmanniae (*Shu Di*), Radix Panacis Ginseng (*Ren Shen*), Radix Astragali Membranacei (*Huang Qi*), Sclerotium Pararadicis Poriae Cocos (*Fu Shen*), Rhizoma Gastrodiae (*Tian Ma*), mix-fried Radix Glycyrrhizae (*Zhi Gan Cao*), Pericarpium Citri Reticulatae (*Chen Pi*), Herba Seu Flos Schizonepetae Tenuifoliae (*Jing Jie*), Radix Ledebouriellae Sesloidis (*Fang Feng*), Radix Et Rhizoma Notopterygii (*Qiang Huo*), Rhizoma Coptidis Chinensis (*Huang Lian*)

4. *Qi Zhen San* (from *Zheng Zhi Zhun Sheng [Patterns & Treatments Norms & Criteria]*): Radix Ligustici Wallichii (*Chuan Xiong*), uncooked Radix Rehmanniae (*Sheng Di*), Herba Cum Radice Asari Seiboldi (*Xi Xin*), Radix Ledebouriellae Sesloidis (*Fang Feng*), Cinnabar (*Zhu Sha*), Rhizoma Acori Graminei (*Shi Chang Pu*), Radix Panacis Ginseng (*Ren Shen*)

5. *Yu Feng Tang:* See Section Four, chapter Six.

6. *Dang Gui San (*from *Quan Sheng Zhi Mi Fang [Whole Life Pointing Out Confusion Formulas]):* Radix Angelicae Sinensis (*Dang Gui*), Herba Seu Flos Schizonepetae Tenuifoliae (*Jing Jie*). Grind into fine powder, decoct with water and wine, and take.

7. *Tian Ma San (*from *Yi Yu Quan Lu (Records of the Entire Realm of Medicine]):* Rhizoma Gastrodiae (*Tian Ma*), Rhizoma Typhonii Gigantei (*Bai Fu Zi*), Rhizoma Arisaematis *Tian Nan Xing*), Buthus Martensis (*Gan Xie*), ginger(-processed) Rhizoma Pinelliae Ternatae (*Ban Xia*). Grind into fine powder and mix with the juice of uncooked Rhizoma Zingiberis (*Sheng Jiang*) and peppermint wine (*Bo He Jiu*). Take 3g each time, at no fixed time.

Section Seven

Postpartum Difficult Defecation
(*Chan Hou Da Bian Nan*)

If, postpartum, eating and drinking are normal but the stools are difficult and bound. This is called *chan hou da bian nan,* postpartum difficult defecation. If severe, there may be no precipitation for many days.

Disease Causes, Disease Mechanisms

This disease's disease cause is mainly postpartum excessive blood loss. Perished blood damages the fluids. The fluids and humors are insufficient. The intestines thus lose their enrichment and moisture. It is also possible for yin to be vacuous and fire exuberant. Fluids and humors are burnt internally. This leads to the arising of loss of moisture of the intestinal tract. Conveyance and transformation are inhibited and the precipitation of the stools is closed, bound, and difficult.

Disease Patterns

Postpartum the stools are closed and bound or are not free- flowing for many days. The skin is dry, eating and drinking are normal, and there is internal heat, a dry mouth, chest and epigastric glomus and fullness, abdominal region distention and pain, a scarlet red tongue with a thin, yellow, slimy coating, and a fine, choppy or fine, rapid pulse.

Treatment

Treatment principles should be based on a consideration of postpartum bodily vacuity, withered blood and dry intestines. One should administer nourishing the blood and moistening the intestines formulas. Externally use *Zhu Dan Ye Mi Jian Dao Fa* (Pig Bile & Boiled Honey Abduction Method). If qi and blood are both vacuous, then use supplementing the qi and nourishing the blood, assisted by moistening the intestines. In patients with good digestion, one can eat plenty of vegetables and various types of meats. Such patients should also drink dilute honey water as a beverage to quickly make their blood effulgent and their fluids sufficient, therefore the stools are automatically freed and smoothed.

Explanation

1. Difficult defecation is one of the most commonly encountered postpartum patterns. It is mostly due to qi and blood, fluids and humors insufficiency. Therefore, treatment using cold, attacking and precipitating medicinals, appropriate in the case of heat constipation, must not be used recklessly or they will lead to the arising of vacuity desertion.

2. If, postpartum, the appetite is good and the digestion is forceful and strong, one can eat a lot of meats and vegetables. Or one can use honey water every day. This enables the fluids and humors to become effulgent and exuberant. Thus the stools open by themselves.

194

Appended Formulas

1. *Ma Ren Wan (*from *Zheng Zhi Zhun Sheng [Patterns & Treatments Norms & Criteria]):* Semen Cannabis Sativae (*Huo Ma Ren*), 30g, bran stir-fried Fructus Citri Seu Ponciri (*Zhi Ke*), 30g, Radix Panacis Ginseng (*Ren Shen*), 30g, Radix Et Rhizoma Rhei (*Da Huang*), 12g. Grind the above medicinals into powder and make into pills with honey. Take 9g each time, 2 times per day on an empty stomach. Wash down with the liquid from dilute rice porridge.

2. *Zi Chang Wu Ren Wan (*from *Shi Yi De Xiao Fang [Generations of Doctors' Effective Formulas]):* Bran stir-fried Semen Pruni Armeniacae (*Xing Ren*), bran stir-fried Semen Pruni Persicae (*Tao Ren*), Semen Biotae Orientalis (*Bai Zi Ren*), Semen Pini (*Song Zi Ren*), Semen Pruni (*Yu Li Ren*), stir-fried Radix Angelicae Sinensis (*Dang Gui*), Exocarpium Citri Erythrocarpae (*Ju Hong*)

3. *Ma Ren Zhou (*from *Ben Shi Fang [Source Materials Formulas]):* Fructus Perillae Frutescentis (*Su Zi*), Semen Cannabis Sativae (*Huo Ma Ren*), equal parts, washed. Grind into fine powder. Use water and grind again. Take 1 bowl and cook into porridge. Divide this into two portions.

4. *Qing Zao Run Chang Tang (*from *Fu Ke Zhong Yi Liao Fa [TCM Gynecology Treatment Methods]):* Uncooked Radix Rehmanniae (*Sheng Di*), Tuber Ophiopogonis Japonicae (*Mai Dong*), Rhizoma Anemarrhenae (*Zhi Mu*), Radix Albus Paeoniae Lactiflorae (*Bai Shao*), honey mix-fried Radix Angelicae Sinensis (*Dang Gui*), Radix Trichosanthis Kirlowii (*Tian Hua Fen*), Radix Et Rhizoma Rhei (*Da Huang*), Tuber Asparagi Cochinensis (*Tian Dong*), Fructus Schizandrae Chinensis (*Wu Wei Zi*)

5. *Ren Ru Yin (*from *Min Jian Fang [Formulas from Among the People]):* If there is postpartum constipation which has not responded to various medicinals and if one cannot speak, drink human breast milk and it will be cured. This can also be taken for senile vacuity closure. Take 1 teacup, 1-2 times per day.

6. *Ba Zhen Tang:* See Section Two, Chapter Five.

7. *Mi Jian Dao Fa* (from *Shang Han Lun [Treatise on Damage Due to Cold]*): If there is binding in the rectum, one can use the boiled honey abduction method or pig bile juice abduction (*i.e.*, suppositories made from these substances).

Section Eight

Postpartum Scanty Lactation (*Chan Hou Ru Ye Guo Shao*)

If after birthing the breast milk is extremely scanty or there is none, this is called scanty lactation (*ru ye guo shao*). It is also called absent lactation (*que ru*).

Disease Causes, Disease Mechanisms

The causes of this disease are divided into two types. 1) Qi and blood congestion and exuberance. There is thus closure and blockage and thus no movement. 2) Scanty blood and qi weakness. Hence there is no milk which can move. The *Fu Ren Da Quan Liang Fang (A Great, Complete [Collection of] Fine Formulas for Women)* says:

> Women's breast milk is transformed from qi and blood. It is possible that it does not move. This is because of qi and blood vacuity weakness and irregularity of the channels and network vessels.

The *Ru Men Shi Qin (Confucian Respect for One's Parents)* also says:

> It is possibly due to wailing, jealousy, and anger to become depressed and bound. This results in the vessels of the breast not moving.

Generally speaking, 8 out of 10 cases of this condition are related to scanty blood and malnutrition (literally, poor construction and nourishment).

Based on clinical experience, the remainder pertain to qi and blood congestion and closure and mental/emotional disturbance (literally, essence spirit stimulation). Treatment must, therefore, take into account these disease causes and be based on their analysis.

Disease Patterns

Qi & Blood Vacuity Weakness

In postpartum women, there is scanty lactation or a total lack of lactation, soft breasts, no breast distention or painful feeling, no discharge of milk or discharge of only a few drops even when the breast is pressed, a somber white facial complexion, essence spirit fatigue, vertigo, dizziness, tinnitus, heart palpitations, possible night sweats, poor appetite, vexatious heat in the five hearts, and facial flushing. The tongue is pale red, and the pulse is fine and weak or fine and rapid.

Liver Qi Depression & Stagnation

Postpartum, the breast milk does not move. There is breast distention, hardness, and pain, chest oppression, hiccup, dual-sided lateral costal distention and pain, no thought for food or drink, head distention, headache, and a wiry pulse.

Treatment

Qi & Blood Vacuity Weakness

One should supplement the qi and nourish the blood. The formula to use is *Jia Wei Si Wu Tang* (Added Flavors Four Materials Decoction). If there is blood vacuity essence spirit fatigue and complete absence of breast milk, one can use *Dang Gui Bu Xue Tang* (Dang Gui Supplement the Blood Decoction) plus Bulbus Allii Fistulosi (*Cong Bai*), 10 stalks. Or *Tong Ru Tang* (Open the Breasts Decoction) or *Zhu Ti Tang* (Pig's Foot Decoction)

197

can also be used. In addition, among the people, *Chi Dou Zhou* (Aduki Bean Porridge) is also commonly used.

Liver Qi Depression & Stagnation

One should soothe the liver and open the breasts. The formula to use is *Tong Gan Sheng Ru Tang* (Open the Liver & Engender Milk Decoction) or *Tong Cao San* (Tetrapanax Powder). If there is breast distention and pain or swelling and pain with lumps, *Luo Lu San* (Echinops Powder) or *Tong Quan San* (Free the Spring Powder) are appropriate. These can be used for treatment following the pattern.

Explanation

1. In women's scanty lactation, if it is due to qi and blood vacuity and debility and construction and nourishment are poor, one must supplement and full the construction and nourishment by eating a lot of such nutritious foods as pig's feet. Thus the breast milk will automatically increase. Not uncommonly, this helps increase lactation even quicker than herbal medication.

2. It is widely known to that one's essence spirit (*i.e.*, mental emotional) state is connected to lactation. If liver/spleen depression, resentment, and anger are not soothed, eventually the breast milk will become diminished and scanty. Intensive inquiry is, therefore, indispensable to the appropriate management of such cases. Treatment for such cases typically includes medicinals for soothing the liver and opening breasts. These should be accompanied by instructions to help quiet her essence spirit.

3. If, due to liver qi depression and binding, the breast milk does not move and there are lumps in the breast, or if there is aversion to cold, fever, and other such symptoms, prompt treatment is necessary in order to prevent mastitis.

Appended Formulas

1. *Jia Wei Si Wu Tang:* Radix Angelicae Sinensis (*Dang Gui*), Radix Ligustici Wallichii (*Chuan Xiong*), stir-fried Radix Albus Paeoniae Lactiflorae (*Bai Shao*), uncooked Radix Rehmanniae (*Sheng Di*), Caulis Akebiae Mutong (*Mu Tong*), Semen Vaccariae Segetalis (*Wang Bu Liu Xing*), Radix Trichosanthis Kirlowii (*Tian Hua Fen*). Boil together with a soup made from pig's feet and take. Before taking this decoction, first use onion soup to wash the nipple and the breast.

2. *Dang Gui Bu Xue Tang:* See Section Two, Chapter Six.

3. *Tong Ru Tang* (from *Jing Yan Fang [Experiential Formulas]*): Pig's Feet (*Zhu Ti*), Medulla Tetrapanacis Papyriferi (*Tong Cao*), Radix Ligustici Wallichii (*Chuan Xiong*), Squama Manitis Pentadactylis (*Chuan Shan Jia*), Radix Glycyrrhizae (*Gan Cao*). Boil the juice and drink.

4. *Zhu Ti Tang* (from *Pao Yun Ji Fang [A Collection of Protecting Pregnancy Formulas]*): Pig's Feet (*Zhu Ti*), 2 pieces, Medulla Tetrapanacis Papyriferi (*Tong Cao*), 60g. First wash the pig's feet and then boil it and the Tetrapanax in water and wine. Afterwards, drink the juice.

5. *Chi Dou Yin* (from *Yi Lue Liu Shu [A Synopsis of Medicine in Six Books]*): Cook roughly ground Semen Phaseoli Calcarati (*Chi Dou*) into porridge and take on an empty stomach.

6. *Tong Gan Sheng Ru Tang* (from *Fu Qing Zhu Nu Ke [Fu Qing-zhu's Gynecology]*): Stir-fried Radix Albus Paeoniae Lactiflorae (*Bai Shao*), Radix Angelicae Sinensis (*Dang Gui*), Rhizoma Atractylodis Macrocephalae (*Bai Zhu*), prepared Radix Rehmanniae (*Shu Di*), Radix Glycyrrhizae (*Gan Cao*), Tuber Ophiopogonis Japonicae (*Mai Dong*), Medulla Tetrapanacis Papyriferi (*Tong Cao*), Radix Bupleuri (*Chai Hu*), Radix Polygalae Tenuifoliae (*Yuan Zhi*)

7. *Tong Cao San:* Radix Platycodi Grandiflori (*Jie Geng*), Tuber Ophiopogonis Japonicae (*Mai Dong*), Radix Bupleuri (*Chai Hu*), Radix

Trichosanthis Kirlowii (*Tian Hua Fen*), Medulla Tetrapanacis Papyriferi (*Tong Cao*), Radix Angelicae Dahuricae (*Bai Zhi*), Radix Rubrus Paeoniae Lactiflorae (*Chi Shao*), Fructus Forsythiae Suspensae (*Lian Qiao*), Caulis Akebiae Mutong (*Mu Tong*), Radix Glycyrrhizae (*Gan Cao*)

8. *Lou Lu San* (from *Yi Lue Liu Shu [A Synopsis of Medicine in Six Books]*): Radix Rubrus Paeoniae Lactiflorae (*Chi Shao*), Radix Platycodi Grandiflori (*Jie Geng*), Radix Angelicae Dahuricae (*Bai Zhi*), Radix Glycyrrhizae (*Gan Cao*), Spina Gleditschiae Chinensis (*Zao Jiao Ci*), Radix Angelicae Sinensis (*Dang Gui*), Radix Ligustici Wallichii (*Chuan Xiong*), Fructus Citri Seu Ponciri (*Zhi Ke*), Radix Saussureae Seu Vladimiriae (*Mu Xiang*)

9. *Tong Quan San*: Semen Vaccariae Segetalis (*Wang Bu Liu Xing*), white Flos Caryophylli (*Bai Ding Xiang*), Radix Rhapontici Seu Echinopsis (*Lou Lu*), Radix Trichosanthis Kirlowii (*Tian Hua Fen*), Bombyx Batryticatus (*Jiang Can*), equal parts. Grind in powder and take 12g each time.

Chapter Eight

Miscellaneous Diseases (*Za Bing*)

In the classification of gynecological disease, menstrual diseases, *dai xia*, and prenatal and postpartum diseases are the main ones. Less important ones are considered miscellaneous diseases or *za bing*. The commonly seen miscellaneous diseases in women are breast *yong* or abscess, uterine prolapse, concretions and conglomerations, accumulations and gatherings (*i.e.*, various types of abdominal masses), plum seed qi, visceral agitation, and infertility.

Breast abscess is caused either by breast milk amassment and accumulation congesting and hindering the milk ducts or by liver depression, anger, and resentment internally frustrating. In general, at the initial stage of its arising, one should clear and scatter. If it is unburst or has already burst, one should support the interior and expel pus. If qi and blood are vacuous and weak and if, after bursting, it does not astringe and restrain (*i.e.*, pull back over) for a long time, one should simultaneously clear heat and supplement the qi and blood.

Uterine prolapse downward desertion is mainly due to qi vacuity falling downward. Therefore, one should mainly upbear and supplement the original qi. If there is liver channel damp heat pouring downward, *Long Dan Xie Gan Tang* (Gentiana Drain the Liver Decoction) treats this.

As for concretions and conglomerations, accumulations and gatherings, concretions and accumulation have form and substance, while conglomerations and gatherings have form but no substance. Food concretion is mainly treated by coursing and abducting. For blood concretion, quicken the blood and dispel stasis. For conglomeration, course the liver and open depression. If the spleen and stomach are vacuous and weak and the qi mechanism is inhibited, treatment should fortify the spleen and rectify the qi.

Plum seed qi is due to susceptibility to anger not being disciplined as well as to worry and thinking or, in other words, internal damage by the seven passions. Visceral agitation is due to heart yin insufficiency and heart fire shining on lung metal above. For this *Gan Mai Da Zao Tang* (Licorice, Wheat & Red Date Decoction) is good.

Infertility is mostly due to kidney qi insufficiency and *chong* and *ren* vacuity cold, liver qi depression and binding, or phlegm dampness obstructing and stagnating. Thus its causes are not all the same and its treatment methods are also consequently variable. If there is kidney vacuity, one should supplement the kidneys and full the essence. If there is liver depression, one should course the liver and resolve depression. If there is blood vacuity, one should nourish the blood and boost the qi. If there is stasis heat, one should transform stasis and clear heat. And if there is phlegm dampness, one should transform phlegm and eliminate dampness. Therefore its treatment should be based on its causes and follow its patterns.

Section One

Breast Abscess (*Ru Yong*)

During the time a woman is breast-feeding, suddenly there may occur breast redness, swelling, and burning pain. The breast milk is reduced and scanty. Simultaneously, there is aversion to cold, fever, and other such generalized symptoms. Several days later, the redness and swelling are followed by pus and ulceration. This is called breast *yong* or abscess.

Disease Causes, Disease Mechanisms

This disease's causes are divided into the two types of internal causes and external causes. Internal causes are *yang ming* and *jue yin* wind heat congesting and exuberant in these two channels. Of this Dan-xi said:

> The breasts are canalized by the *yang ming*; the *jue yin* homes to the

nipples. If the birthing woman is not harmonious, regular, and nourished, if resentment and anger cause counterflow, or if preference for thick flavors result in depression and oppression, the *jue yin* qi does not move. Thus the portals are not open and free-flowing and the breast milk cannot obtain exit. *Yang ming* heat boils and seethes and this heat therefore transforms pus. Its external cause is due to damage of the breast by exposure to wind or the suckling infant's mouth blowing. Breast milk amasses and accumulates and does not flow smoothly. This causes swelling and pain and the creation of breast *yong*.

The *Chao Shi Bing Yuan (Master Chao's Source of Disease)* says:

Hot food and sweating damage of the breast by exposure to wind, these produce susceptibility to breast swelling, and each can produce blowing breasts.

The *Yi Xue Xin Wu (Heart Realizations in the Study of Medicine)* also says:

When the infant suckles, the infant blows its mouth qi. This results in the breast milk not being free-flowing. It congests and becomes stagnant and there is swelling and pain. If not treated immediately, it becomes *yong*.

As these quotations state, in terms of the disease causes of breast abscess, the internal causes have to do with essence spirit depression and binding, worry, thought, resentment, and anger. Thus the breast is not free-flowing. In terms of the external causes, they are hot food and sweating, damage of the breath due to exposure to wind, and the suckling infant's mouth qi.

Disease Patterns

Initial Stage Exterior Pattern Breast Abscess

The breast milk is not free-flowing and there is amassment and accumulation internally. The breasts are aching and painful, swollen and distended. There is congestion and blockage of the milk ducts. There are, due to occlusion of the mammary ducts, palpable lumps and pressure increases the pain. The exterior of the breast is red and swollen. There is bodily cold, fever, headache, chest oppression, aching and pain of the bones and joints, and no sweating. The tongue coating is superficial and white. The pulse is floating and tight or floating and rapid. This is evils in the exterior. If there is redness, swelling, and slight pain, no dizziness, and a dry mouth, this is the normal flow (*i.e.*, progression of this disease). If the pulse is surging and rapid and the tongue coating is excessive and yellow, there is evil heat but the righteous is exuberant. There is smoldering and brewing, rottening and transformation. This also produces pus and blood.

Suppurative Stage Breast Abscess

Bodily cold and fever have already resolved. The breast swelling has diminished and feels soft. The skin in the affected area is red, there is aching and pain, and there is about to be bursting. If the abscess has already burst, then there is ulceration with thick, yellow pus. The swelling disperses and the pain then stops. If it proceeds normally, the area around the lesion becomes itchy and new flesh is engendered. If there are multiple ulcers with heart vexation, vomiting, and no eating, this is a contrary development. If there is a ruptured ulcer whose meat is purplish black colored, pain radiating to the heart, and an emaciated, weak body, this mostly is categorized as dying of the righteous.

Qi & Blood Vacuity Breast Abscess

The facial complexion is somber white. There is essence spirit fatigue, a pronounced desire to sleep, breast pain which is mild, swelling and hardness like a stone which is difficult to burst, and a vacuous, weak, fine pulse.

Treatment

Initial Stage Exterior Pattern Breast Abscess

One should relieve the exterior, disperse and scatter. Internally one should take *Jing Fang Niu Bang Tang* (Schizonepeta, Ledebouriella & Arctium Decoction) combined with *Lian Qiao Jin Bei Jian* (Forsythia, Lonicera & Fritillaria Decoction). However, if there is breast swelling and pain but absence of bodily cold, fever, and other such symptoms of an exterior pattern, one can use *Shen Xiao Gua Lou San* (Spirit-like Effect Trichosanthes Powder). If Spica Prunellae Vulgaris (*Xia Ku Cao*) and Pericarpium Viridis Citri Reticulatae (*Qing Pi*) are added, the effect is even better. If there is also qi and blood vacuity weakness, one should also use qi and blood supplementing medicinals at the same time. Or one can use *Xing Xiao Wan* (Arouse & Disperse Pills). In addition, no matter if there is no exterior pattern, one should simultaneously use an externally applied treatment. Where there is breast aching and pain, externally use *Chan Su Ding* (Toad Secretion Lozenge) mixed with vinegar. Or one can use *Cong Yun Fa* (Onion Ironing Method) in order to aid dispersion and scattering and to avoid the transformation of pus.

Suppurative Stage Breast Abscess

If the swelling becomes soft and there is local brightness of the skin, heat, redness, aching and pain, pus has already formed, and the lesion is about to burst or has burst and is discharging a thick, yellow, pussy fluid, one should use surgery to cut open and expel the pus. Or one can use *Shen Xiao Gua Luo San* (Spirit-like Effect Trichosanthes Powder) plus Squama Manitis Pentadactylae (*Chuan Shan Jia*), Radix Codonopsis Pilosulae (*Dang Shen*), and Radix Astragali Membranacei (*Huang Qi*). Or one can use *Tuo Li Xiao Du San* (Support the Interior & Disperse Toxins Powder) plus Squama Manitis Pentadactylis (*Chuan Shan Jia*). Externally one can apply *Shen Xian Tai Yi Gao* (Spirit Immortal *Tai Yi* Paste).

Qi & Blood Vacuity Breast Abscess

If there is breast abscess which is swollen, hard, difficult to burst, and the pain is relatively mild, one can use *Tuo Li Xiao Du San* (Support the Interior & Disperse Toxins Powder). After bursting, if the pussy fluid is clear and watery and endures for many days without closing, one should warm and supplement the qi and blood. One can use *Yi Qi Yang Rong Tang* (Boost the Qi & Nourish the Constructive Decoction) or *Tuo Li Xiao Du San* (Support the Interior & Disperse Toxins Powder) minus Flos Lonicerae Japonicae (*Jin Yin Hua*) and Spina Gleditschiae Chinensis (*Zao Jiao Ci*) but with double doses of Radix Panacis Ginseng (*Shen*), Radix Astragali

205

Membranacei (*Qi*) or plus Radix Lateralis Praeparatus Aconiti Carmichaeli (*Fu Zi*).

Explanation

1. The *Feng Shi Jin Nang (Master Feng's Wise Counsel)* describes various approaches for the comprehensive treatment of breast abscess:

> If there is breast abscess in the initial stage with aversion to cold and fever, the breast is red, swollen, and burning hot, then one should emit the exterior and scatter evils, course the liver and clear stomach heat, speedily precipitate the breast milk, and abduct the congestion and blockage. Then the disease must be cured. If not scattered, it will easily become a *yong* or abscess. Then it is appropriate to support the interior and disperse toxins. If, after it has burst, flesh is not engendered and there is pussy water which is clear and runny, one should supplement the spleen and stomach. If pus exits from the skin of *yong* and there is aversion to cold and fever, one should regulate the constructive and defensive. If there is heat, swelling, and pain when breast-feeding, one should supplement yin and blood. If the appetite is scanty and there is vomiting, one should supplement the stomach qi. Cold, cool, toxin-resolving medicinals are, in that case, prohibited since they might further damage the spleen and stomach.

The above quotation is cited for the reader's reference. Its principles should be used flexibly, taking into consideration all the bodily symptoms, the cause of the onset of the disease, and treating based on the pattern.

2. Breast abscess is mostly seen in primiparas. In order to prevent breast abscess, it is essential that the breasts be kept clean and warm. One should not let the newborn sleep with the nipple in its mouth. Each time after suckling at night, one should express any remaining milk so that congestion and accumulation may not produce disease. It is also important to protect the good cheer of one's essence spirit.

3. This disease is mostly engendered in breast-feeding women, but clinically, it may also be seen in women who are not breast-feeding. However, their number is small. This is mostly due to essence spirit depression and binding from worry, thinking, resentment, and anger being

206

greatly excessive. Internal heat congests and binds and thus leads to its arising.

Appended Formulas

1. *Jing Fang Niu Bang Tang (*from *Yi Zong Jin Jian [Golden Mirror of Ancestral Medicine]):* Herba Seu Flos Schizonepetae Tenuifoliae (*Jing Jie*), Radix Ledebouriellae Sesloidis (*Fang Feng*), stir-fried Fructus Arctii (*Niu Bang Zi*), Flos Lonicerae Japonicae (*Jin Yin Hua*), Pericarpium Citri Reticulatae (*Chen Pi*), Radix Trichosanthis Kirlowii (*Tian Hua Fen*), Radix Scutellariae Baicalensis (*Huang Qin*), Herba Cum Radice Taraxaci Mongolici (*Pu Gong Ying*), Fructus Forsythiae Suspensae (*Lian Qiao*), Spina Gleditschiae Chinensis (*Zao Jiao Ci*), Radix Bupleuri (*Chai Hu*), Rhizoma Cyperi Rotundi (*Xiang Fu*), Radix Glycyrrhizae (*Gan Cao*)

2. *Lian Qiao Jin Bei Jian (*from *Jing Yue Quan Shu (Jing-yue's Complete Writings]):* Flos Lonicerae Japonicae (*Jin Yin Hua*), Bulbus Fritillariae Thunbergii (*Zhe Bei Mu*), Herba Cum Radice Taraxaci Mongolici (*Pu Gong Ying*), Spica Prunellae Vulgaris (*Xia Ku Cao*), Caulis Sargentodoxae (*Hong Teng*), Fructus Forsythiae Suspensae (*Lian Qiao*)

3. *Shen Xiao Gua Luo San (*from *Wai Ke Ji Yan Fang [Collected Proven Formulas in External Medicine]):* Fructus Trichosanthis Kirlowii (*Gua Lou*), Radix Glycyrrhizae (*Gan Cao*), Radix Angelicae Sinensis (*Dang Gui*), Resina Olibani (*Ru Xiang*), Resina Myrrhae (*Mo Yao*). Decoct in water and remove the dregs. Add 1 teacup of aged wine, divide into 3 doses, and take after eating.

4. *Xing Xiao Wan (*from *Tai Ping Hui Min He Ji Ju Fang [Tai Ping Imperial Grace Formulary]):* Processed Resina Olibani (*Ru Xiang*), processed Resina Myrrha (*Mo Yao*), Realgar (*Xiong Huang*), Secretio Moschi Moschiferi (*She Xiang*). Each time take 9g washed down with hot aged wine. The patient is then asked to go to bed completely covered by quilts to induce perspiration. The swelling will have dispersed and the pain will have stopped when the patient awakens from her alcoholic intoxication.

5. *Tuo Li Xiao Du San (*from *Yi Zong Jin Jian [Golden Mirror of Ancestral Medicine])*: Radix Panacis Ginseng (*Ren Shen*), Radix Astragali Membranacei (*Huang Qi*), Spina Gleditschiae Chinensis (*Zao Jiao Ci*), Radix Platycodi Grandiflori (*Jie Geng*)

6. *Yi Qi Yang Rong Tang (*from *Zheng Zhi Zhun Sheng [Patterns & Treatments Norms & Criteria])*: Radix Panacis Ginseng (*Ren Shen*, Sclerotium Poriae Cocos (*Fu Ling*), Pericarpium Citri Reticulatae (*Chen Pi*), Bulbus Fritillariae Thunbergii (*Zhe Bei Mu*), Radix Angelicae Sinensis (*Dang Gui*), Radix Ligustici Wallichii (*Chuan Xiong*), Radix Astragali Membranacei (*Huang Qi*), prepared Radix Rehmanniae (*Shu Di*), stir-fried Radix Albus Paeoniae Lactiflorae (*Bai Shao*), Radix Platycodi Grandiflori (*Jie Geng*), Radix Glycyrrhizae (*Gan Cao*), Rhizoma Atractylodis Macrocephalae (*Bai Zhu*), Radix Bupleuri (*Chai Hu*)

7. *Chan Su Ding (*from *Yang Yi Da Quan [A Great, Complete {Collection of} Ulcer Medicine])*: Secretio Bufo Bufonis (*Chan Su*) dissolved in wine, mix-fried Resina Myrrhae (*Mo Yao*), mix-fried Resina Olibani (*Ru Xiang*), Realgar (*Xiong Huang*), defatted Semen Crotonis Tiglii (*Ba Dou Shuang*), Camphora (*Nao Sha)*, Cinnabar (*Zhu Sha*), Secretio Moschi Moschiferi (*She Xiang*). Grind these into powder and make into pills the size of mung beans using the Secretio Bufo Bufonis dissolved in wine. Each time, use 1 pill, applied to the local area, and covered with a plaster.

8. *Cong Yun Fa:* Apply mashed green onions with roots on the affected area of the breast and cover with a jar in which there is a smoldering piece of charcoal. Leave in place until the patient begins to perspire profusely. Then withdraw.

Section Two

Uterine Prolapse (*Yin Ting*)

Uterine prolapse (is also called uterine desertion and heaviness (*zi gong tuo zhong*). The degrees of pressure of the uterine descension and heaviness are not the same. It can divided into grade 1, grade 2, and grade 3. Grade 1 refers to the dropping of the cervix below the horizontal level of the protuberance of the sitz bone. However, it does not desert and exit from the mouth of the vaginal tract. Grade 2 refers to the uterine cervix and part of the uterus deserting and exiting from the mouth of the vaginal tract on the outside. And grade 3 refers to the total desertion and discharge of the body of the uterus outside the mouth of the vaginal tract.

Disease Causes, Disease Mechanisms

In terms of the causes of this disease, many cases are due to the use of excessive force during parturition or to difficult birth of excessively long duration. It may also be due to postpartum getting up too early and excessive taxation and activity. Further, it may be due to lifting heavy objects, bedroom taxation, and standing too long at one's post before delivery. Constipation, qi vacuity falling downward with inability to secure and contain, and spleen/stomach depressive heat with damp heat pouring downward may all also cause the uterus to desert and exit. However, its main cause is due to qi vacuity not containing. First there is qi vacuity as the main cause. This then results in the above various types of causes and thus the production of this disease.

Disease Patterns

Predominant Qi Vacuity

In one type, there is sudden onset of pressure and heaviness in the lower abdomen, uterine desertion and exiting, radiating pain, nausea, and vomiting. In another type, there slow development of a heavy, sagging sensation in the lower part of the lower abdomen. This leads to a feeling of sagging and dropping in the abdominal region radiating to and causing aching and pain in the sacrum. Eventually, a tumor-like substance deserts and exits from outside the vaginal meatus. Such uterine prolapse typically only occurs in women who work standing up. After the initial dropping, the exposed uterus may become enlarged and impede the normal functions of the bladder and rectum. Commonly this leads to the arising of urinary frequency or anuria, non-free flowing stools or diarrhea. The face is a somber white, the body fears cold, and the essence spirit is fatigued. There are heart palpitations, shortness of breath, a pale tongue with a thin coating, and a vacuous, weak or vacuous, large, forceless pulse.

Predominant Blood Vacuity

There is uterine desertion and exiting. If prolonged, this leads to the manifestation of qi vacuity with blood vacuity signs. There is a sallow yellow facial complexion, dry, parched skin, tinnitus, blurred vision, low back soreness, upper back stiffness, and dry stools. The tongue is pale, and the pulse is vacuous and fine.

Liver Channel Damp Heat

There is uterine desertion and exiting, sort of painful, sort of itching, heart vexation, internal heat, possible generalized heat and spontaneous perspiration, a bitter taste in the mouth, dry throat, chest oppression, torpid intake, scanty sleep at night, constipation, and hot, red urination or frequent, numerous, astringent, and painful urination. The tongue coating is yellow and slimy, and the pulse is slippery and rapid. If there is blood vacuity mixed with dampness, bloody water dribbles and drips and there is a sallow yellow facial complexion, withered, emaciated bodily flesh, vertigo, heart palpitations, burning heat in the hearts of the hands, a fresh red tongue, and a fine, rapid pulse.

Treatment

Predominant Qi Vacuity

One should supplement the center and boost the qi. The formula to use is *Bu Zhong Yi Qi Tang* (Supplement the Center & Boost the Qi Decoction) plus Fructus Citri Seu Ponciri (*Zhi Ke*). If there is blood vacuity, add Gelatinum Corii Asini (*E Jiao*), wine(-processed) Radix Albus Paeoniae Lactiflorae (*Bai Shao*), and Radix Ligustici Wallichii (*Chuan Xiong*). If qi vacuity is mixed with damp heat, add Fructus Gardeniae Jasminoidis (*Zhi Zi*), Sclerotium Poriae Cocos (*Fu Ling*), and Pericarpium Viridis Citri Reticulatae (*Qing Pi*).

Predominant Blood Vacuity

The formula to use is *Shi Quan Da Bu Tang Jia Jian* (Ten [Ingredients] Greatly & Completely Supplementing Decoction with Additions & Subtractions).

Liver Channel Damp Heat

If there is urinary astringency and pain, use *Long Dan Xie Gan Tang* (Gentiana Drain the Liver Decoction). If there is blood vacuity mixed with dampness and bloody water dribbling and dripping, use *Gui Pi Tang Jia Jian* (Restore the Spleen Decoction with Additions & Subtractions). This can be aided by the use of external medicinals: Fructus Cnidii Monnieri (*She Chuang Zi*) and Fructus Pruni Mume (*Wu Mei*) are decocted and used as a fumigation and wash.

Explanation

Although uterine prolapse is not a life-threatening disease, however it can have serious effects on one's work, activities, and strength. In general, when this disease is of short duration, it is easily treated. During the time of treatment, a lot of quiet bed rest heralds a better prognosis. One half year after being healed, one should pay attention not to climb heights, lift heavy objects, indulge in bedroom affairs, overtax oneself, or be too active or these will lead to recurrence. For those with grade 2 or worse desertion heaviness with a protracted disease course, achieving effective treatment is difficult. Therefore, one can use surgery.

2. In this disease, a better effect may be attained by combining with acupuncture treatment. Choose *Guan Yuan* (CV 4), *Qi Hai* (CV 6), *Gui Lai*

(St 29), and *San Yin Jiao* (Sp 6). After needling, moxa.

3. Preventive measures include 1) family planning, 2) care to prevent tearing of the perineum during delivery, 3) prompt repair of any such tears, 4) avoidance of too early resumption of physical labor, and 5) active treatment of chronic diseases such as cough and constipation.

Appended Formulas

1. *Bu Zhong Yi Qi Tang:* See Section One, Chapter Four.

2. *Shi Quan Da Bu Tang:* See section Five, Chapter Four.

3. *Long Dan Xie Gan Tang (*from *Tai Ping Hui Min He Ji Ju Fang [Tai Ping Imperial Grace Formulary]):* Radix Gentianae Scabrae (*Long Dan Cao*), Rhizoma Alismatis (*Ze Xie*), Fructus Gardeniae Jasminoidis (*Zhi Zi*), Radix Scutellariae Baicalensis (*Huang Qin*), uncooked Radix Rehmanniae (*Sheng Di*), Semen Plantaginis (*Che Qian Zi*), Caulis Akebiae Mutong (*Mu Tong*), Radix Glycyrrhizae (*Gan Cao*), Radix Angelicae Sinensis (*Dang Gui*), Radix Bupleuri (*Chai Hu*)

4. *Gui Pi Tang:* See Section One, Chapter Four.

5. The decoction of Fructus Cnidii Monnieri (*She Chuang Zi*) and Fructus Pruni Mume (*Wu Mei*) for fumigating and washing consists of: Fructus Cnidii Monnieri (*She Chuang Zi*), 1 *jin*, Fructus Pruni Mume (*Wu Mei*), 14 pieces. Boil the above medicinals into a decoction. Wash the prolapsed uterus several times each evening.

6. *Zhen Hui Tang Jing Yan Fang* (True Kindness Hall Empirical Formula): Fructus Citri Seu Ponciri (*Zhi Ke*), 2 *liang*. Boil into a decoction and soak and wash with this.

7. *Luo Shi Hui Yue Yi Jin Fang* (Master Luo's Skillful, Economical, Medical Brocade Formula): Fructus Citri Seu Ponciri (*Zhi Ke*), Fructus

212

Terminaliae Chebulae (*He Zi*), Fructus Schizandrae Chinensis (*Wu Wei Zi*), Alum (*Bai Fan*). Boil into a decoction and fumigate and wash. If not astringed moxa *Bai Hui* (GV 20) at the top of the head several cones.

8. *Xun Xi Fang* (Fumigation & Washing Formula): Herba Seu Flos Schizonepetae Tenuifoliae (*Jing Jie*), Cortex Ailanthi Altissimi (*Chun Gen Pi*), Folium Agastachis Seu Pogostemi (*Huo Xiang Ye*). Boil into a decoction and fumigate and wash.

9. *Cha Yao* (Application Medicinals): First wash with a decoction of Radix Lophatheri Gracilis (*Dan Zhu Gen*). Then use Galla Rhi Chinensis (*Wu Bei Zi*) and Alum (*Bai Fan*) ground into powder. Apply.

Section Three

Concretions & Conglomerations, Accumulations & Gatherings (*Zheng Jia Ji Ju*)

Concretions and conglomerations, accumulations and gatherings are a type of disease pattern which refers to bound lumps within the abdomen. These may be accompanied by fullness, distention, or pain. They may be secure and immovable, or they may be occasional and movable. Sometimes they may gather and sometimes they may scatter. Concretions are solid, hard, and difficult to break. They are firm and secure (*i.e.*, have definable borders), and they do not shift around. Their pain is fixed and they are like a hard lump. Thus they are called concretions. Conglomerations make use of materials to produce form. If pushed, they shift, turn, and move. Sometimes they gather and sometimes they scatter. Thus they are called conglomerations. Accumulations are the same as concretions. Generally speaking, accumulations are located in the five viscera. Thus there are five types of accumulations. They pertain to blood disease. Gatherings are the same as conglomerations. Generally speaking, gatherings are located in the six bowels. Thus there are six types of gatherings. They pertain to qi

213

disease. Though this disease may occur in both men and women, they are most often found in the lower abdomens of women due to their particular physiology.

Disease Causes, Disease Mechanisms

The range of disease causes of concretions and conglomerations, accumulations and gatherings is very broad and complex. The *Zhu Bing Yuan Hou Lun (Treatise on the Origins & Symptoms of Various Diseases)* analyzes these in terms of accumulations and gatherings, elusive mass disease, *shan* conglomerations, and concretion glomus. The *Yi Zong Jin Jian (Golden Mirror of Ancestral Medicine)* divides this into food concretions, blood concretions, glomus concretions, accumulations and gatherings, static blood, blood *gu*, and elusive mass *shan* types. In terms of disease causes, the typically seen concretion diseases are food concretions and blood concretions, these two types. The causes of blood concretions are described by Zhang Jing-yue:

> Static blood is retained and stagnates and eventually becomes concretion. Only women have this. This pattern may be due to the menstrual period or postpartum. Internal damage may engender chill or there may be external contraction of wind cold. Anger may damage the liver. Qi counterflows and blood is retained. Or worry and thinking may damage the spleen. Qi becomes vacuous and blood stagnates.

As said, during the menstrual movement and postpartum, surplus blood may not be completely eliminated or one may have counterflow which leads to retention and stagnation. For days this accumulates and slowly this produces concretion. In terms of the production of food concretion, Jing-yue says:

> If food and drink are retained and gather, this produces concretion and glomus or it may be due to the raw, chilled foods, wind cold, resentment and anger with qi counterflow, taxation and fatigue, hunger and satiation, undisciplined eating and drinking. All of these are able to produce it.

214

In terms of the causes of production of conglomerations, the *Fu Ren Da Quan Liang Fang (A Great, Complete [Collection of] Fine Formulas for Women)* says:

> Women's *shan* conglomeration is due to undisciplined eating and drinking, unregulated cold and warmth, qi and blood taxation and damage, viscera and bowel vacuity weakness, wind chill entering the abdomen and mutually binding with the blood. Thus it is engendered.

Based on these statements, concretion and conglomerations, accumulations and gatherings are mainly produced by viscera and bowel vacuity weakness, qi and blood taxation and damage, recent birth, menstrual movement, and not knowing how to be prudent in terms of raw and chilled food and drink, jealousy, anger, worry, and thinking. These lead to damage and hence the production of this condition. This explication of the disease causes and disease mechanisms of this pattern is based on the commonly used terms of former peoples' of food concretions, blood concretions, qi glomus, static blood/blood *gu*, *xuan* elusive mass, *shan* conglomeration, intestinal *tan*, and stone conglomeration, and the differentiation of each of these is presented below.

Disease Patterns

Food Concretion

There are accumulations and lumps in the epigastrium and abdomen which are firm and secure and which do not shift or move. These concretions and lumps slowly grow larger. Following the qi upward and downward, they attack with growing aching and pain. This pain does not like pressure. The desire for food is devitalized. The face is yellow and the flesh is emaciated. There is chest and epigastric distention and fullness, acid eructation, belching and vomiting, and excessively loose stool or constipation. The lips and tongue are lusterless and the tongue coating is thick and turbid. The pulse is deep and choppy.

Blood Concretion

Within the abdomen there are concretions and lumps. They are firm and secure and do not shift. There is lateral costal and abdominal distention and fullness and aching and pain which refuses pressure. Eating food leads to distention, pain, and discomfort within the abdomen. There is bitter pain in both lateral costal regions, perspiration from the region of the head, heart chaos, depression, and oppression, vexation and agitation, fright mania, interior heat with chilled limbs, a yellow face and emaciated, weak flesh and body, a dark, purple tongue, and a *chi* or foot pulse which is surging and rapid.

Qi Glomus

There is chest and diaphragmatic glomus and oppression, qi depression which is not smooth flowing, qi lumps beneath the lateral costal region, and bowstring-like tension and piercing pain. Eating chilled foods causes the onset of aching and pain. When the stomach and epigastrium are satiated, there is oppression and discomfort. The desire for food is devitalized. The tongue coating is thin and white, and the pulse is wiry and choppy.

Static Blood/Blood *Gu*

In women, the menstrual movement static blood ceases and is retained. There is navel abdominal region concretions and lumps. These are firm and secure and do not shift. There is distention, fullness, tension, and pain and no desire for pressure or rubbing. the body is constantly hot or there is tidal fever in the afternoon. The facial complexion is a sallow yellow. If brewing and accumulation endure for many days, the menstrual water is not free-flowing and this produces blood *gu* disease. The tongue is purple and dark, and the pulse is choppy.

Xuan Elusive Mass

In women, sinews on both sides of the navel on the abdomen protrude. There is uncommon aching and pain. The size of the protrusion may be as large as a fist to as small as a finger. Its form may be like bowstring which is tight and hard. Or it may be located between the ribs. When there is pain, one can see it. When there is no pain, it is not there. The tongue coating is thin and white, and the pulse is wiry and choppy.

Shan Conglomeration

In women, there may be attacking, surging, piercing pain in the lower abdomen which may radiate to the low back and lateral costal regions. Severe pain may be felt during paroxysmal attack when obvious protrusion of the lower abdomen can be seen. When there is no pain, the abdomen is normal looking. There is also frequent, numerous urination, inhibited urination, or abnormal vaginal discharge. The tongue coating is thin, and the pulse is wiry and urgent or choppy.

Intestinal *Tan*, Stone Conglomeration

Within the abdomen there are concretions and lumps. These may be as large as a chicken egg. Each day they slowly increase in size until it is as if the woman were pregnant. When pressed, they are hard and they are difficult to shift. If the menstruation continues to come each month, this is intestinal *tan*. If the menstruation is blocked and stops, this is stone conglomeration.

Treatment

Food Concretion

For women's food concretion, if there are accumulations and lumps within the abdomen which do not disperse and the body is still strong and replete, one should mainly course and abduct. Use *Wu Yao San* (Lindera Powder) or *Da Qi Qi Tang* (Major Seven Qi Decoction). If the body is weak and the period of disease relatively protracted, if the woman's spleen and stomach are vacuous and weak, or if the desire for food is devitalized, use *Liu Jun Zi Tang* (Six Gentlemen Decoction) and externally apply *E Wei Gao* (Asafoetida Paste).

217

Blood Concretion

If a woman has a lump within her abdomen which is disc-like, firm, and unshifting, her menstruation does not move, and there is bodily fatigue, one should mainly use *Xue Jie San* (Dragon's Blood Powder). If there is mental oppression, fright, and mania with a surging, rapid pulse, add *Da Quan Fang*(Great Complete Formula) in order to dispel blood stasis. Then mania and agitation will automatically stop.

Qi Glomus

If there is chest and diaphragmatic glomus and oppression with qi depression which does not diffuse, mainly use *Zhu Qi Wan* (Assist the Qi Pills). If there is phlegm rheum, food accumulation, and depression and oppression, use *Kai Yu Zheng Yuan San* (Open Depression & Correct the Origin Powder). If their spleen and stomach are not fortified and the body is weak and the qi is vacuous, one can use *Xiang Sha Lui Jun Zi Tang* (Saussurea & Amomum Six Gentlemen Decoction) to fortify the spleen and rectify the qi.

Static Blood, Blood *Gu*

If women have static blood ceasing and retained with lumps and pain around the their navel in the abdomen or the lochia does not move, use *Shi Xiao San* (Sudden Smile Powder) to dispel malign blood. If the menses are closed and not free-flowing and static blood congeals and gathers, one can use *Tao Nu San* (Immature Fructus Persicae Powder). If the person's body is fatigued, if there is little thought for food or drink, the disease has endured for many days, and the body's qi is all insufficient, one should use *Liu Jun Zi Tang* (Six Gentlemen Decoction), possibly adding Radix Ligustici Wallichii (*Chuan Xiong*), Radix Angelicae Sinensis (*Dang Gui*), blast-fried Rhizoma Zingiberis (*Pao Jiang*), and Cortex Cinnamomi (*Rou Gui*) to warm and supplement.

Xuan Elusive Mass

If a woman has *xuan* elusive mass with protrusion on both sides of her navel giving rise to aching and pain, use *Cong Bai San* (Allium Fistulosum Powder) to warm and scatter. Or one can use *Wu Ji Jian Wan* (Black Chicken Decoction Pills) taken at the same time for better effect.

Shan Conglomeration

If a woman has lower abdominal attacking, surging, piercing pain radiating to the low back and lateral costal regions with evident protruding mass, one should use *Dang Gui San* (Dang Gui Powder) or *Pan Cong San* (Curled Onion Powder) to warm the stomach, free the flow of the network vessels, and dispel stasis.

Intestinal *Tan*, Stone Conglomeration

For intestinal *tan*, use *Er Chen Tang* (Two Aged [Ingredients] Decoction) plus Rhizoma Cyperi Rotundi (*Xiang Fu*) to open this. Or one can use *Shi Jin Mo Fang* (Execute Modern Learning Decoction) or *Wu Hui Wan* (Black Snout Pills) to disperse and scatter. If there is stone conglomeration pattern with blocked, stopped menstruation, use *Jian Xian Dan* (Evidence Showing Elixir) to attack and dispel.

Explanation

Women with concretions and conglomerations, accumulations and gatherings are commonly encountered in clinical practice. Treatment should take into account not only intensive inspection and inquiry regarding the patient's general strength and exuberance, debility and weakness, whether the disease is new or enduring, and its history, but should also take into account the patient's reaction to any previous therapy or treatments she may have received. Otherwise, mismanagement of such cases by recklessly administering attacking formulas is likely to damage the patient's righteous qi and may even endanger her life destiny. The *Ji Yin*

219

Gang Mu (Detailed Outline of Yin) says:

> Proper treatment of concretions and conglomerations regulates the qi and breaks the blood, disperses food and cracks phlegm. However, when the size is reduced by half, stop. It is not all right to violently attack and harshly execute or this will damage the original qi. Rather, support the spleen and stomach righteous qi and wait for it to be spontaneously transformed.

The *Yi Zong Jin Jian (Golden Mirror of Ancestral Medicine)* also says:

> The classic says, great accumulation, great gathering, it is all right to attack this. Once it is debilitated by half, stop for fear that excessive attacking will damage the qi and blood.

The formulas discussed in this section for the treatment of the various patterns of this disease are primarily composed of many attacking medicinals. In clinical practice, those with enduring disease usually have vacuous weak bodies. Therefore, paying attention to the righteous qi, it is preferable to combine attacking with supplementation. Once the righteous qi is sufficient, the effect and force of attacking medicinals is amplified and one can achieve victory all the quicker.

Appended Formulas

1. *Wu Yao San (*from *Fu Ren Da Quan Liang Fang [A Great, Complete [Collection of} Fine Formulas for Women]):* Radix Linderae Strychnifoliae (*Wu Yao*), Rhizoma Curcumae Zedoariae (*E Zhu*), Cortex Cinnamomi (*Rou Gui*), Radix Angelicae Sinensis (*Dang Gui*), Semen Pruni Persicae (*Tao Ren*), Pericarpium Viridis Citri Reticulatae (*Qing Pi*), Radix Saussureae Seu Vladimiriae (*Mu Xiang*). Grind into powder, mix with hot wine, and down, 6g each time.

2. *Da Qi Qi Tang (*form *Ji Sheng Fang [Formulas for the Aid of the Living]):* Rhizoma Sparganii (*San Leng*), Rhizoma Curcumae Zedoariae (*E Zhu*), Pericarpium Viridis Citri Reticulatae (*Qing Pi*), Pericarpium Citri Reticulatae (*Chen Pi*), Radix Saussureae Seu Vladimiriae (*Mu Xiang*),

Fructus Alpiniae Oxyphyllae (*Yi Zhi Ren*), Radix Platycodi Grandiflori (*Jie Geng*), Cortex Cinnamomi (*Rou Gui*), mix-fried Radix Glycyrrhizae (*Zhi Gan Cao*)

3. *Liu Jun Zi Tang* (from *Tai Ping Hui Min He Ji Ju Fang [Tai Ping Imperial Grace Formulary]*): Radix Panacis Ginseng (*Ren Shen*), Sclerotium Poriae Cocos (*Fu Ling*), Rhizoma Atractylodis Macrocephalae (*Bai Zhu*), Radix Glycyrrhizae (*Gan Cao*), Rhizoma Pinelliae Ternatae (*Ban Xia*), Pericarpium Citri Reticulatae (*Chen Pi*)

4. *E Wei Gao* (from *Su Shi Liang Fang [Master Su's Fine Formulas]*): Radix Et Rhizoma Notopterygii (*Qiang Huo*), Radix Angelicae Pubescentis (*Du Huo*), Radix Scrophulariae Ningpoensis (*Xuan Shen*), Cortex Cinnamomi (*Rou Gui*), Radix Rubrus Paeoniae Lactiflorae (*Chi Shao*), Squama Manitis Pentadactylis (*Chuan Shan Jia*), uncooked Radix Rehmanniae (*Sheng Di*), Radix Et Rhizoma Rhei (*Da Huang*), Radix Angelicae Dahuricae (*Bai Zhi*, Rhizoma Gastrodiae (*Tian Ma*), Rhizoma Anemonis Raddeanae (*Liang Tou Jian*), 15g each; Flos Carthami Tinctorii (*Hong Hua*), Ramulus Sophorae Japonica (*Huai Tiao*), Ramulus Pruni Persicae (*Tao Zhi*), 9g each; Semen Momordicae Cochinensis (*Mu Bei Zi*), 10 pieces without the skin; Human Hair (*Luan Fa*), amount like 3 chicken eggs. Use 2 *jin* 4 *liang* of fragrant oil (*i.e.*, roasted sesame seed oil [*Xiang You*]), boil till black, and remove the dregs. Then aid the hair and boil. When the hair has almost dissolved, remove the dregs. Then add Minium (*Huang Dan*) and cook until it becomes a soft, plastic consistency. Then add Mirabilitum (*Mang Xiao*), Resina Ferulae Asafoetidae (*E Wei*), Styrax Oil (*Su He Xiang You*), Resina Olibani (*Ru Xiang*), and Resina Myrrhae (*Mo Yao*), 15g each. Finally mix in some Secretio Moschi Moschiferi (*She Xiang*) and the paste is made. Spread this paste on the affected area.

5. *Xue Jie San:* Sanguis Draconis (*Xue Jie*), Radix Angelicae Sinensis (*Dang Gui*), Radix Rubrus Paeoniae Lactiflorae (*Chi Shao*), Pollen Typhae (*Pu Huang*), Rhizoma Corydalis Yanhusuo (*Yan Hu Suo*)

6. *Da Quan Fang:* Semen Pruni Persicae (*Tao Ren*), Feces Trogopterori Seu Pteromi (*Wu Ling Zhi*), uncooked Radix Rehmanniae (*Sheng Di*),

Radix Achyranthis Bidentatae (*Niu Xi*), Radix Et Rhizoma Rhei (*Da Huang*), Radix Glycyrrhizae (*Gan Cao*)

7. *Zhu Qi Wan* (from *Shen Shi Zhun Sheng Shu* [*Master Shen's Writings on Respecting Life*])*:* Rhizoma Sparganii (*San Leng*), Rhizoma Curcumae Zedoariae (*E Zhu*). Wrap in wet paper, bake, and cut into slices, 480g each. Pericarpium Viridis Citri Reticulatae (*Qing Pi*), Pericarpium Citri Reticulatae (*Chen Pi*), Rhizoma Atractylodis Macrocephalae (*Bai Zhu*), 225g each; bran stir-fried Fructus Citri Seu Ponciri (*Zhi Ke*), Semen Arecae Catechu (*Bing Lang*), Radix Saussureae Seu Vladimiriae (*Mu Xiang*), 150g each. Powder all of the above and make into pills. Take 9g each time washed down with warm water.

8. *Kai Yu Zheng Yuan San* (from *Ji Yin Gang Mu* [*Detailed Outline of Yin*])*:* Rhizoma Atractylodis Macrocephalae (*Bai Zhu*), Pericarpium Citri Reticulatae (*Chen Pi*), Pericarpium Viridis Citri Reticulatae (*Qing Pi*), Rhizoma Cyperi rotundi (*Xiang Fu*), Fructus Crataegi (*Shan Zha Rou*), Radix Platycodi Grandiflori (*Jie Geng*), Sclerotium Poriae Cocos (*Fu Ling*), Fructus Amomi (*Sha Ren*), Rhizoma Corydalis Yanhusuo (*Yan Hu Suo*), stir-fried Massa Medica Fermentata (*Shen Qu*), stir-fried Fructus Germinatus Hordei Vulgaris (*Mai Ya*), mix-fried Radix Glycyrrhizae (*Zhi Gan Cao*), uncooked Rhizoma Zingiberis (*Sheng Jiang*)

9. *Xiang Sha Liu Jun Zi Tang:* See Section Two, Chapter Four.

10. *Shi Xiao San:* See Section Ten, Chapter Four.

11. *Tao Nu San:* Stir-fried Fructus Immaturus Pruni Persicae (*Tao Nu*), stir-fried Feces Ratti Norvegici (*Shu Fen*), Rhizoma Corydalis Yanhusuo (*Yan Hu Suo*), Fructus Amomi (*Sha Ren*), Semen Pruni Persicae (*Tao Ren*). Powder the above medicinals and take 9g each time mixed with warm wine.

12. *Liu Jun Zi Tang Jia Xiong Gui:* Radix Panacis Ginseng (*Ren Shen*), clerotium Poriae Cocos (*Fu Ling*), Rhizoma Atractylodis Macrocephalae (*Bai Zhu*), mix-fried Radix Glycyrrhizae (*Zhi Gan Cao*), Rhizoma Pinelliae

Ternatae (*Ban Xia*), Pericarpium Citri Reticulatae (*Chen Pi*), Radix Ligustici Wallichii (*Chuan Xiong*), Radix Angelicae Sinensis (*Dang Gui*), blast-fried Rhizoma Zingiberis (*Pao Jiang*), Cortex Cinnamomi (*Rou Gui*)

13. *Cong Bai San (*from *Zheng Zhi Zhun Sheng [Patterns & Treatments Norms & Criteria]):* Caulis Alli Fistulosi (*Lian Ti Cong Bai*), Radix Ligustici Wallichii (*Chuan Xiong*), Radix Angelicae Sinensis (*Dang Gui*), Fructus Citri Seu Ponciri (*Zhi Ke*), Cortex Magnoliae Officinalis (*Hou Po*), Cortex Cinnamomi (*Rou Gui*), dry Rhizoma Zingiberis (*Gan Jiang*), Fructus Foeniculi Vulgaris (*Hui Xiang*), Radix Albus Paeoniae Lactiflorae (*Bai Shao*), Pericarpium Viridis Citri Reticulatae (*Qing Pi*), Radix Saussureae Seu Vladimiriae (*Mu Xiang*), Fructus Germinatus Hordei Vulgaris (*Mai Ya*), Rhizoma Sparganii (*San Leng*), Rhizoma Curcumae Zedoariae (*E Zhu*), Fructus Meliae Toosendan (*Chuan Lian Zi*), Sclerotium Poriae Cocos (*Fu Ling*), Massa Medica Fermentata (*Shen Qu*), Radix Panacis Ginseng (*Ren Shen*), prepared Radix Rehmanniae (*Shu Di*)

14. *Wu Ji Jian Wan (*from *Tai Ping Hui Min He Ji Ju Fang [Tai Ping Imperial Grace Formulary]):* Take 9g each time with warm wine on an empty stomach.

15. *Dang Gui San (*from *Zheng Zhi Zhun Sheng [Patterns & Treatments Norms & Criteria]):* Radix Angelicae Sinensis (*Dang Gui*), Radix Ligustici Wallichii (*Chuan Xiong*), Carapax Amydae Sinénsis (*Bei Jia*), Fructus Evodiae Rutecarpae (*Wu Zhu Yu*), Semen Pruni Persicae (*Tao Ren*), Radix Rubrus Paeoniae Lactiflorae (*Chi Shao*), Cortex Cinnamomi (*Rou Gui*), Semen Arecae Catechu (*Bing Lang*), Pericarpium Viridis Citri Reticulatae (*Qing Pi*), Radix Saussureae Seu Vladimiriae (*Mu Xiang*), Rhizoma Curcumae Zedoariae (*E Zhu*), Radix Et Rhizoma Rhei (*Da Huang*)

16. *Pan Cong San (*from *Tai Ping Hui Min He Ji Ju Fang [Tai Ping Imperial Grace formulary]):* Rhizoma Corydalis Yanhusuo (*Yan Hu Suo*), Cortex Cinnamomi (*Rou Gui*), dry Rhizoma Zingiberis (*Gan Jiang*), Radix Glycyrrhizae (*Gan Cao*), Rhizoma Atractylodis (*Cang Zhu*), Fructus Amomi (*Sha Ren*), Cortex Caryophylli (*Ding Xiang Pi*), Semen Arecae (*Bing Lang*), Rhizoma Curcumae Zedoariae (*E Zhu*), Rhizoma Sparganii (*San*

223

Leng), Sclerotium Poriae Cocos (*Fu Ling*), Pericarpium Viridis Citri Reticulatae (*Qing Pi*). Powder the above medicinals and take 9g each time.

17. *Er Chen Tang Jia Xiang Fu:* See Section One, Chapter Six, to which should be added Rhizoma Cyperi Rotundi (*Xiang Fu*).

18. *Shi Jin Mo Fang:* Semen Citri Reticulatae (*Ju He*), Radix Albus Paeoniae Lactiflorae (*Bai Shao*), Radix Bupleuri (*Chai Hu*), carbonized Folium Artemisiae Argyii (*Ai Ye*), Gelatinum Corii Asini (*E Jiao*), Radix Ligustici Wallichii (*Chuan Xiong*), Radix Angelicae Sinensis (*Dang Gui*), prepared Radix Rehmanniae (*Shu Di*), Rhizoma Corydalis Yanhusuo (*Yan Hu Suo*), Rhizoma Atractylodis (*Cang Zhu*), Cortex Phellodendri (*huang Bai*), mix-fried Radix Glycyrrhizae (*Zhi Gan Cao*), Thallus Algae (*Kun Bu*), boiled in water, Fructus Meliae Toosendan (*Chuan Lian Zi*), stir-fried with 3g of Semen Crotonis Tiglii (*Ba Dou*), after stir-frying, remove the Croton Seeds, prepared Radix Rehmanniae (*Shu Di*), pounded with Fructus Amomi (*Sha Ren*), do not remove the Amomum.

19. *Wu Hui Wan:* Radix Aconiti (*Wu Tou*), blast-fry and remove the skin, Rhizoma Pinelliae Ternatae (*Ban Xia*), calcined Gypsum Fibrosum (*Shi Gao*), stir-fried Herba Veratri Nigri (*Li Lu*), Concha Ostreae (*Mu Li*), Sclerotium Poriae Cocos (*Fu Ling*), Cortex Cinnamomi (*Rou Gui*), dry Rhizoma Zingiberis (*Gan Jiang*), Semen Crotonis Tiglii (*Ba Dou*). Grind the above medicinals into powder and make into pills with honey the size of mung bans. Take 3-5 pills each time, drunk with wine after meals.

20. *Jian Xian Dan (*from *Wei Sheng Bao Jian [The Precious Mirror of Defending Life]):* Blast-fried Radix Lateralis Praeparatus Aconiti Carmichaeli (*Fu Zi*), Herba Buchnerae Cruciatae (*Gui Jian Yu*), Fluoritum (*Zi Shi*), Rhizoma Alismatis (*Ze Xie*), Cortex Cinnamomi (*Rou Gui*), Rhizoma Corydalis Yanhusuo (*Yan Hu Suo*), Radix Saussureae Seu Vladimiriae (*Mu Xiang*), Sanguis Draconis (*Xue Jie*), Hirudo (*Shui Zhi*), Semen Arecae Catechu (*Bing Lang*), Semen Pruni Persicae (*Tao Ren*), Rhizoma Sparganii (*San Leng*), Rhizoma Curcumae Zedoariae (*E Zhu*), Radix Et Rhizoma Rhei (*Da Huang*). Grind the above into fine powder and make pills with wine. Wash down with vinegar soup or warm wine. Take before meals.

Section Four

Plum Seed Qi (*Mei He Qi*)

In the *Jin Gui Yao Lue (Essentials from the Golden Cabinet)*, plum seed qi is called *zhi rou*, roasted meat. It refers to the disease where women feel phlegm in their throats similar to roasted meat which can neither be swallowed down nor spit out. Although men can also have this disease, it is relatively seldom seen.

Disease Causes, Disease Mechanisms

In terms of the causes of this disease, the *Qian Jin Fang (Thousand [Pieces of] Gold Formulas)* says, "Internal damage by the seven passions, external damage by cold cause it." You Zai-jing says, "This is congealed phlegm binding with qi which obstruct and blocks the throat." Based on these sayings, its causes are susceptibility to anger which is undisciplined, worry and thinking, plus other damages of the seven passions. These result in the visceral qi becoming depressed and bound. Phlegm drool and qi mutually wrestle and counterflow upward to the throat where they produce this disease.

Disease Patterns

Predominant Heat

Within the throat there is phlegm drool obstructing and blocking. It can neither be swallowed down nor spit out. There is dry throat and a bitter taste in the mouth, heart vexation, restlessness, dry, parched stools, a thin tongue coating, and a wiry, rapid pulse.

Predominant Cold

Within the throat there is phlegm drool obstructing and blocking. Swallowing or spitting it are difficult. There may also be nausea, vomiting, a lusterless facial complexion, a slimy, white tongue coating, and a slippery, relaxed (*i.e.*, retarded) pulse image.

Treatment

Predominant Heat

One should resolve depression and clear heat. The formula to use is *Dan Zhi Xiao Yao San* (Moutan & Gardenia Rambling Powder).

Predominant Cold

One should scatter binding and diffuse the qi. The formula to use is *Ban Xia Hou Po Tang* (Pinellia & Magnolia Decoction).

Explanation

The cause of plum seed qi is phlegm and qi mutually obstructing. "Phlegm congeals and binds with qi which obstructs and blocks the throat." *Ban Xia Hou Po Tang* (Pinellia & Magnolia Decoction) opens phlegm and descends qi. This is truly effective for treating this disease. However, in many people, this disease is due to thinking and worry, depression and binding. Therefore, Dan-xi's *Yue Ju Wan* (Escape Restraint Pills) should also be considered for use.

Appended Formulas

1. *Dan Zhi Xiao Yao San:* See Section Two, Chapter Six.

2. *Ban Xia Hou Pu Tang (*from *Jin Gui Yao Lue [Essentials from the Golden Cabinet]):* Rhizoma Pinelliae Ternatae (*Ban Xia*), Cortex Magnoliae Officinalis (*Hou Po*), Sclerotium Poriae Cocos (*Fu Ling*), uncooked Rhizoma Zingiberis (*Sheng Jiang*), Folium Perillae Frutescentis (*Zi Su*)

Section Five

Visceral Agitation (*Zang Zao*)

Women may be damaged by sorrow for no reason. They may weep and smile without constancy. Later they may act like a normal person. This kind of disease is called visceral agitation. The *Jing Gui Yao Lue (Essentials from the Golden Cabinet)* says:

> Women's visceral agitation — joy and sorrow distress one and they desire to cry. They are as if possessed by a spirit. They also yawn many times. *Gan Mai Da Zao Tang* (Licorice, Wheat & Red Date Decoction) rules this.

Correctly this refers to this disease.

Disease Causes, Disease Mechanisms

The cause of this disease is mainly heart construction insufficiency and heart fire upward dazzling lung metal. The heart rules joy and the lungs rule sorrow. The heart produces smiles and the lungs produce crying. Therefore, there is distress due to sorrow and deep grief, crying and smiling with no constancy. The kidneys rule yawning. If heart yin is already vacuous, heart fire is hyperactive above and is not able to descend and join with the kidneys. Thus there is much yawning and stretching.

Disease Patterns

This disease may come at any time. Those who have it are sorrowful for no reason and cry and smile without constancy. Afterwards they return to being like a normal person. Sometimes they eat a lot and sometimes little. At night they may sleep, they may be addicted to lying down, or they may not sleep. There may be constant sighing, yawning, and stretching the lower back. The stools may be constipated. The tongue is red with a scanty coating. The tongue may be peeled bare and have cracks and fissures. The pulse is wiry and rapid. It is also possible that there is spiritual fatigue, heart palpitations, shortness of breath, heart vexation, fright and watchfulness (*i.e.*, paranoia), internal heat and a dry mouth, a red tongue, and a fine, rapid pulse.

Treatment

One should mainly use *Gan Mai Da Zao Tang* (Licorice, Wheat & Red Date Decoction). If there are heart palpitations, shortness of breath, internal heat, a dry mouth, then add to the above formula *Dan Zhu Ru Tang* (Bland Caulis Bambusae Decoction). If there is abdominal pain, add to the above formula Radix Albus Paeoniae Lactiflorae (*Bai Shao*). If there is no vexation and irritation or desire to cry, then remove Fructus Zizyphi Jujubae (*Da Zao*) from the above formula and add uncooked Radix Rehmanniae (*Sheng Di*), Fructus Hordei Vulgaris (*Mai Ya*), Gelatinum Corii Asini (*E Jiao*), uncooked Os Draconis (*Long Gu*), and Egg Yolk (*Ji Zi Huang*).

Explanation

The treatment of this disease can be combined with acupuncture/moxibustion. Mainly choose the point *Nei Guan* (Per 6). Needles should be inserted bilaterally and retained for from 30 minutes to 1 hour. The effects of this are extremely good.

Appended Formulas

1. *Gan Mai Da Zao Tang* (from *Jin Gui Yao Lue [Essentials from the Golden Cabinet])*: Mix-fried Radix Glycyrrhizae (*Zhi Gan Cao*), Fructus Levis Tritici Aestivi (*Xiao Mai*), Fructus Zizyphi Jujubae (*Da Zao*)

2. *Dan Zhu Ru Tang* (from *Chan Ke Xin Fa [Obstetrical Heart Methods])*: Radix Panacis Ginseng (*Ren Shen*), Sclerotium Poriae Cocos (*Fu Ling*), Rhizoma Pinelliae Ternatae (*Ban Xia*), Tuber Ophiopogonis Japonicae (*Mai Dong*), Radix Glycyrrhizae (*Gan Cao*), Caulis In Taeniis Bambusae

(*Zhu Ru*), uncooked Rhizoma Zingiberis (*Sheng Jiang*), Fructus Zizyphi Jujubae (*Da Zao*)

Section Six

Infertility (*Bu Yun Zheng*)

Infertility refers to a married woman not being able to conceive after over 3 years even though both parties are healthy or failure to conceive for several years after already conceiving at least one child. This is called *bu yun*, infertility.

Disease Causes, Disease Mechanisms

there are many causes of infertility. It may be due to physiological defects, such as the so-called five not females (*wu bu nu*): *luo* or spiral, *wen* or atresia, *gu* or drum, *jiao* or horn, and *mai* or sterility (*i.e.*, types of congenital malformation of the genitalia.) Pathologically, the causes of infertility are kidney vacuity, uterine cold, blood vacuity, liver depression, stasis heat, and phlegm dampness, these six types.

Disease Patterns

Kidney Vacuity

There is no conception after several years of marriage. The menses are late and scanty in amount. The color of the menstruate is dark (*i.e.*, dull) and pale. Or the menses may be blocked and not move. There is low back soreness as if about to snap, dizziness, tinnitus, a chilly feeling in the lower abdomen, loose stools, long, clear urination, a dark, dull facial complexion, a pale tongue with a thin, white coating, and a deep, fine, forceless pulse.

Uterine Cold

There is a prolonged menstrual discharge, scant in volume, dark, blackish in color, chilly pain in the lower abdomen which diminishes when it obtains heat, a thin, white tongue coating, and a deep, slow pulse.

Blood Vacuity

There is a sallow yellow facial complexion, late menstruation which is scanty in amount and pale in color, dizziness, vertigo, dry, parched skin, constipation, insidious pain in the lower abdomen after menstruation, a pale tongue, and a fine, weak pulse.

Liver Depression

There is early or late menstruation which is scanty in volume and dark red in color, lower abdominal distention and pain, premenstrual breast distention and pain, essence spirit depression, eructation, and sighing. The tongue coating is thin, and the pulse is wiry.

Stasis Heat

There is scanty menstrual volume which is purplish red in color and contains clots. There is lower abdominal distention and pain, especially along the sides, which refuses pressure, bodily emaciation, a long history of low back soreness, chest and lateral costal distention and pain. The tongue is red with a thin coating. The pulse is wiry and rapid.

Phlegm Dampness

There is bodily obesity, a history of excessive phlegm, a somber white facial complexion, possible superficial edema, delayed menstruation or amenorrhea, and excessive vaginal discharge. The tongue has a thin, white coating, and the pulse is wiry and slippery.

Treatment

Kidney Vacuity

One should supplement the kidneys and warm the essence, warm and nourish the uterus. The formula to use is *Yu Lin Zhu* (Fostering Unicorn Pearls), *You Gui Wan* (Restore the Right [Kidney] Pills), or *Wu Zi Yan Zong Wan* (Five Seeds Spread Out the Ancestors Pills).

Uterine Cold

One should warm the uterus and scatter cold. The formula to use is *Ai Fu Nuan Gong Wan* (Artemisia & Cyperus Warm the Palace Pills).

Blood Vacuity

One should supplement the blood and boost the qi. The formula to use is *Ren Shen Yang Rong Tang* (Ginseng Nourish the Constructive Decoction) or *Yang Jing Zhong Yu Tang* (Nourish the Essence Jade Seed Decoction). In case of severe anemia, add Cornu Cervi (*Lu Jiao Pian*) and Placenta Hominis (*Zi He Che*) to fill the essence and transform the blood.

Liver Depression

One should course the liver and resolve depression. The formula to use is *Chai Hu Shu Gan San* (Bupleurum Course the Liver Powder) or *Kai Yu Zhong Yu Tang* (Open Depression Jade Seed Decoction). If there is breast distention and pain, add Tuber Curcumae (*Yu Jin*) and Fructus Akebiae (*Ba Yue Zha*). For lumps, add Semen Citri Reticulatae (*Ju He*), Fructus Liquidambaris Taiwaniae (*Lu Lu Tong*), and Squama Manitis Pentadactylis (*Chuan Shan Jia*). If there is heat, add Cortex Radicis Moutan (*Dan Pi*) and Fructus Gardeniae Jasminoidis (*Shan Zhi*).

Stasis Heat

One should clear the heat and transform stasis. The formula to use is *Qing*

231

Re Xiao Yu Tang (Clear Heat & Disperse Stasis Decoction).

Phlegm Dampness

One should fortify the spleen and transform dampness, rectify the qi and transform phlegm. The formula to use is *Xiao Zhi Mo Dao Tan Tang* (Disperse Fatty Tissue & Abduct Phlegm Decoction) or *Qi Gong Wan* (Open the Palace Pills).

Explanation

1. Determination of the cause of infertility requires examination of both the man and woman, including gynecological examination of the female and physical examination and sperm examination of the male.

2. Clinically, the most commonly seen patterns of infertility are kidney vacuity and liver depression. Therefore, the main treatment principles are to supplement the kidneys and fill the essence, course the liver and resolve depression.

3. For the maldevelopment of the uterus and ovarian insufficiency, routine treatment often consists of *You Gui Wan* (Restore the Right [Kidney] Pills), *Wu Zi Yan Zong Wan* (Five Seeds Spread the Ancestors Pills), or other such prescriptions to which Gelatinum Cornu Cervi (*Lu Jiao Jiao*) and Placenta Hominis (*Zi He Che*) are added in order to aid the growth of the uterus and facilitate ovarian function by supplementing the kidneys and strengthening yang, nourishing the essence and boosting the blood.

4. During treatment for infertility, the patient should be instructed to arrange her sexual activity so as to seize the right moment of ovulation to ensure the goal of impregnation.

Appended Formulas

1. *Yu Lin Zhu* (from *Jing Yue Quan Shu [Jing Yue's Complete Writings]*): Radix Panacis Ginseng (*Ren Shen*), Rhizoma Atractylodis Macrocephalae

232

(*Bai Zhu*), Sclerotium Poriae Cocos (*Fu Ling*), wine stir-fried Radix Albus Paeoniae Lactiflorae (*Bai Shao*), mix-fried Radix Glycyrrhizae (*Zhi Gan Cao*), Radix Angelicae Sinensis (*Dang Gui*), prepared Radix Rehmanniae (*Shu Di*), processed Semen Cuscutae (*Tu Si Zi*), wine stir-fried Cortex Eucommiae Ulmoidis (*Du Zhong*), Cornu Degelatinum Cervi (*Lu Jiao Shuang*), Fructus Zanthoxyli Bungeani (*Chuan Jiao*), Radix Ligustici Wallichii (*Chuan Xiong*)

2. *You Gui Wan:* See Section Ten, Chapter Four.

3. *Wu Zi Yan Zhong Wan (*from *Zheng Zhi Zhun Sheng [Patterns & Treatments Norms & Criteria]):* Semen Cuscutae (*Tu si Zi*), Fructus Schizandrae Chinensis (*Wu Wei Zi*), Fructus Lycii Chinensis (*Gou Qi Zi*), Fructus Rubi (*Fu Pen Zi*), Semen Plantaginis (*Che Qian Zi*)

4. *Ai Fu Nuan Gong Wan (*from *Shen Shi Zun Sheng Shu [Master Shen's Writings on Respecting Life]):* Folium Artemisiae Argyii (*Ai Ye*), Rhizoma Cyperi Rotundi (*Xiang Fu*), Radix Angelicae Sinensis (*Dang Gui*), Radix Dipsaci (*Xu Duan*), Fructus Corni Officinalis (*Shan Zhu Yu*), Radix Ligustici Wallichii (*Chuan Xiong*), Radix Albus Paeoniae Lactiflorae (*Bai Shao*), Radix Astragali Membranacei (*Huang Qi*), prepared Radix Rehmanniae (*Shu Di*), Cortex Cinnamomi (*Rou Gui*)

5. *Ren Shen Yang Rong Tang:* See Section Two, Chapter Four.

6. *Yang Jing Zhong Yu Tang (*from *Fu Qing Zhu Nu Ke [Fu Qing-zhu's Gynecology]):* Prepared Radix Rehmanniae (*Shu Di*), wine stir-fried Radix Angelicae Sinensis (*Dang Gui*), wine stir-fried Radix Albus Paeoniae Lactiflorae (*Bai Shao*), prepared Fructus Corni Officinalis (*Shan Zhu Yu*)

7. *Chai Hu Shu Gan San (*from *Jing Yue Quan Shu [Jing-yue's Complete Writings]):* Pericarpium Citri Reticulatae (*Chen Pi*), Radix Bupleuri (*Chai Hu*), Radix Albus Paeoniae Lactiflorae (*Bai Shao*), Fructus Citri Seu Ponciri (*Zhi Ke*), mix-fried Radix Glycyrrhizae (*Zhi Gan Cao*), Radix Ligustici Wallichii (*Chuan Xiong*), Rhizoma Cyperi Rotundi (*Xiang Fu*)

8. *Kai Yu Zhong Yu Tang (*from *Fu Qing Zhu Nu Ke [Fu Qing-zhu's Gynecology]):* Wine stir-fried Radix Albus Paeoniae Lactiflorae (*Bai Shao*), wine stir-fried Rhizoma Cyperi Rotundi (*Xiang Fu*), wine stir-fried Radix Angelicae Sinensis (*Dang Gui*), earth stir-fried Rhizoma Atractylodis Macrocephalae (*Bai Zhu*), wine stir-fried Cortex Radicis Moutan (*Dan Pi*), Sclerotium Poriae Cocos (*Fu Ling*), Radix Trichosanthis Kirlowii (*Hua Fen*)

9. *Qing Re Xiao Yu Tang (*from *Ben Yuan Jing Yan Fang [Capital Bureau Experiential Formulas]):* Radix Angelicae Sinensis (*Dang Gui*), scorched Radix Albus Paeoniae Lactiflorae (*Bai Shao*), Fructus Meliae Toosendan (*Chuan Lian Zi*), Radix Bupleuri (*Chai Hu*), Caulis Sargentodoxae (*Hong Teng*), Rhizoma Corydalis Yanhusuo (*Yan Hu Suo*), stir-fried Fructus Citri Seu Ponciri (*Zhi Ke*), Tuber Curcumae (*Yu Jin*), *Ji Su San* (Chicken Reviving Powder, *i.e.,* Talcum [*Hua Shi*], Radix Glycyrrhizae [*Gan Cao*], Herba Menthae Haplocalysis [*Bo He*])

10. *Xiao Zhi Mo Dao Tan Tang (*from *Ji Yin Gang Mu [Detailed Outline of Yin]):* Processed Rhizoma Pinelliae Ternatae (*Ban Xia*), processed Rhizoma Arisaematis (*Nan Xing*), Exocarpium Citri Erythrocarpae (*Ju Hong*), Fructus Citri Seu Ponciri (*Zhi Ke*), Sclerotium Poriae Cocos (*Fu Ling*), Talcum (*Hua Shi*), Radix Ligustici Wallichii (*Chuan Xiong*), Radix Ledebouriellae Sesloidis (*Fang Feng*), Radix Et Rhizoma Notopterygii (*Qiang Huo*), Semen Plantaginis (*Che Qian Zi*)

11. *Qi Gong Wan (*from *Jing Yan Fang [Experiential Formulas]):* Rhizoma Atractylodis (*Cang Zhu*), processed Rhizoma Pinelliae Ternatae (*Ban Xia*), Sclerotium Poriae Cocos (*Fu Ling*), infant urine stir-fried Rhizoma Cyperi Rotundi (*Xiang Fu*), stir-fried Massa Medica Fermentata (*Shen Qu*), Pericarpium Citri Reticulatae (*Chen Pi*), Radix Ligustici Wallichii (*Chuan Xiong*)

Index

A

abdomen, aching and pain in the 54
abdomen, attacking, surging, piercing pain in the lower 217
abdomen, insidious pain in the lower 48, 53, 230
abdomen, sinews on both sides of the navel on the, protrude 217
abdominal aching and pain, sudden lower 165
abdominal distention, fullness, and panting 148
abdominal distention, occasional 69
abdominal distention, pain, and discomfort, very faint lower 52
abdominal fullness 122, 149, 150, 171
abdominal masses 201
abdominal pain during pregnancy 121, 122, 125
abdominal pain, occasional 129
abdominal pain, postpartum 164-167
abdominal pain which likes pressure 44, 140, 170, 173
abdominal pain which refuses pressure 140, 183
abdominal region distention and pain 194
abdominal region, empty pain in the 170
abdominal region, sagging and dropping in the 209
abdominal region, soft 173
abortion, threatened 149
abscess, breast 23, 201-207
accumulations and gatherings 201, 213, 219
acupuncture 6, 112, 211
acupuncture and moxibustion 7, 112
acupuncture, reckless 112
agitation 69, 76, 84, 166, 184, 201, 202, 216, 218, 227
amenorrhea 9, 11, 25, 47, 66, 67, 230
anger, easy 61, 65, 84, 85, 123, 135
aphasia 176, 177, 190, 191
appetite, devitalized 41, 68, 135
appetite, picky 114, 115
appetite, poor 31, 35, 41, 197
appetite, scanty 77, 86

B

back and abdominal soreness and pain, low 135
back and knee soreness and stiffness, low 127
back and knee soreness and weakness, low 29, 42, 48, 78, 85, 159, 183
back region, soreness in the low 5
back pain, severe low 94
back pain, upper 69, 84
back soreness, low 36, 54, 68, 69, 77, 84-86, 93, 96, 106, 118, 126, 128, 134, 136, 140, 142, 144, 150, 182, 210, 229, 230
back soreness as if about to snap, low 229
back soreness, long history of low 230
back soreness, lower and upper 40, 54, 94
bao luo 1, 12, 57
bao mai 1, 13, 52, 53, 68, 76, 121, 164
bao tai 2, 4, 147
basal body temperature 103
bedroom affairs 9, 26, 27, 40, 42, 44, 52, 90, 92, 95, 96, 112, 142, 143, 211
bedroom taxation 22, 47, 67, 71, 76, 127, 163, 209
belching 29, 41, 115, 122, 128, 215
belching and burping 122, 128
Ben Shi Fang 72, 157, 195
Ben Yuan Jing Yan Fang 234
beng lou 74, 80, 81
Bian Chan Xu He 112
Bing Yu Tang Yan Fang 97
birth diseases, before 109
birth, early 139
birth mat period 163
birth, small 127, 139-144
births, too many 76
bleeding, mid-cycle 103
blood concretion 201, 216, 218
blood pressure, high 84, 156
blood *gu* 214-216, 218
blood, vanquished 140, 171, 177, 191
body, cold 30, 94, 110, 122, 135, 169, 203, 204
body, cold, and chilled limbs 94
bone pain 182
bones and joints, aching and pain of the 122, 204

brain disease 156
breast abscess 23, 201-206
breast diseases 23
breast distention 5, 11, 25, 35, 40, 53, 64, 66, 110, 183, 197, 198, 230-231
breast distention, hardness, and pain 197
breast, pain in the 65
breast *yong* 13, 201-203
breasts, burning heat in the 65
breasts, enlargement of the 5
breasts, soft 197
breath, shortness of 35, 41, 46, 69, 77, 86, 122, 149, 155, 159, 173, 210, 228
breathing, asthmatic 149
Bu Yi Fang 132

C

Chan Bao 38, 152
Chan Bao Bai Wen 38
Chao Shi Bing Yuan 203
cheeks, flushed red 61
cheeks, occasional red 155
Chen Zi-ming 4
chest and diaphragmatic inhibition 135
chest and diaphragmatic satiation and oppression 183
chest and epigastric fullness and oppression 48, 155, 179
chest and epigastric glomus and fullness 194
chest and epigastric satiation and oppression 122
chest and lateral costal distention and oppression 65, 101
chest and lateral costal or breast distention and pain 41, 53
chest oppression 30, 35, 69, 76, 118, 160, 171, 173, 197, 203, 210
chill, fear of 30, 86, 149, 159, 173, 183
chill, fear of, by the lower extremities 149
chong and *ren* 2, 3, 9-12, 15, 17, 19, 20, 22, 25, 28, 29, 34, 39-42, 44, 45, 47, 48, 53, 68, 75, 76, 85, 90, 127, 140, 163, 170, 172, 202
chong and *ren,* detriment and damage of the 11, 7
chong mai 2-4, 9, 11, 17, 19, 84, 85
clots 5, 26, 29, 35, 48, 53, 56, 57, 77, 173, 183, 230

cold and heat coming alternately 183
cold, aversion to 8, 35, 68, 121, 123, 174, 182, 183, 198, 202, 206
cold, fear of 78, 85, 128, 166, 190
concretion, blood 201, 216, 218
concretion, food 201, 215, 216, 218
concretions and conglomerations 10, 11, 70, 201, 213, 214, 219, 220
concretions and lumps, navel abdominal region 217
conglomeration, *shan* 215-217, 219
conglomeration, stone 216, 218, 220
consciousness of human affairs, lack of 154
constipation 6, 44, 77, 85, 118, 122, 155, 179, 183-185, 194, 195, 209, 210, 212, 215, 230
convulsive seizures 189
cough 69, 122, 182, 212
counterflow 13, 60, 61, 114-117, 149, 171, 175, 190, 203, 214, 225
crying and smiling with no constancy 227

D

Da Sheng Yao Zhi 120
dai mai 3, 9, 12, 23, 89-91, 93, 100, 105
dai xia 21, 89-93, 96, 100, 104, 106, 144, 201
dai xia, watery 144
Dan Xi Xin Fa 28, 31, 92, 99
defecating numerous times 135
defecation, difficult 13, 163, 193, 194
depression and oppression 13, 203, 218
depression, emotional 25, 28, 29, 34, 65, 68, 101
desire for both warmth and pressure 53
desire for heat and fear of cold 128
diarrhea 128, 160, 183, 210
dietary therapy 119
distention and pain which does not desire pressure 53
dizziness 5, 6, 22, 29, 30, 35, 40, 41, 44, 46, 48, 52, 54, 65, 68, 69, 76, 77, 84-86, 89, 110, 115, 122, 127, 135, 140, 142, 144, 149, 150, 154-156, 159, 163, 165, 169, 173, 176-180, 182, 183, 197, 204, 229
dizziness and vertigo 29, 30, 76, 89
downward sagging and discomfort 122
dreams, erotic 90
dribbling and dripping without stop 41

241

OTHER BOOKS ON CHINESE MEDICINE AVAILABLE FROM BLUE POPPY PRESS

3450 Penrose Place, Suite 110, Boulder, CO 80301
For ordering 1-800-487-9296 PH. 303\447-8372 FAX 303\245-8362

A NEW AMERICAN ACUPUNC-TURE by Mark Seem, ISBN 0-936185-44-9

ACUPOINT POCKET REFERENCE ISBN 0-936185-93-7

ACUPUNCTURE AND MOXI-BUSTION FORMULAS & TREATMENTS by Cheng Dan-an, trans. by Wu Ming, ISBN 0-936185-68-6

ACUTE ABDOMINAL SYN-DROMES: Their Diagnosis & Treatment by Combined Chinese-Western Medicine by Alon Marcus, ISBN 0-936185-31-7

AGING & BLOOD STASIS: A New Approach to TCM Geriatrics by Yan De-xin, ISBN 0-936185-63-5

AIDS & ITS TREATMENT ACCORDING TO TRADITIONAL CHINESE MEDICINE by Huang Bing-shan, trans. by Fu-Di & Bob Flaws, ISBN 0-936185-28-7

BETTER BREAST HEALTH NATURALLY with CHINESE MEDICINE by Honora Lee Wolfe & Bob Flaws ISBN 0-936185-90-2

THE BOOK OF JOOK: Chinese Medicinal Porridges, An Alterna-tive to the Typical Western Break-fast by B. Flaws, ISBN0-936185-60-0

CHINESE MEDICAL PALMIS-TRY: Your Health in Your Hand by Zong Xiao-fan & Gary Liscum, ISBN 0-936185-64-3

CHINESE MEDICINAL TEAS: Simple, Proven, Folk Formulas for Common Diseases & Promoting Health by Zong Xiao-fan & Gary Liscum, ISBN 0-936185-76-7

CHINESE MEDICINAL WINES & ELIXIRS by Bob Flaws, ISBN 0-936185-58-9

CHINESE PEDIATRIC MAS-SAGE THERAPY: A Parent's & Practitioner's Guide to the Prevention & Treatment of Childhood Illness by Fan Ya-li, ISBN 0-936185-54-6

CHINESE SELF-MASSAGE THERAPY: The Easy Way to Health by Fan Ya-li ISBN 0-936185-74-0

A COMPENDIUM OF TCM PAT-TERNS & TREATMENTS by Bob Flaws & Daniel Finney, ISBN 0-936185-70-8

CURING ARTHRITIS NATURALLY WITH CHINESE MEDICINE by Douglas Frank & Bob Flaws ISBN 0-936185-87-2

CURING DEPRESSION NATURALLY WITH CHINESE MEDICINE by Rosa Schnyer & Bob Flaws ISBN 0-936185-94-5

CURING HAY FEVER NATURALLY WITH CHINESE MEDICINE by Bob Flaws, ISBN 0-936185-91-0

CURING INSOMNIA NATURALLY WITH CHINESE MEDICINE by Bob Flaws ISBN 0-936185-85-6

CURING PMS NATURALLY WITH CHINESE MEDICINE by Bob Flaws ISBN 0-936185-85-6

THE DAO OF INCREASING LONGEVITY AND CONSERVING ONE'S LIFE by Anna Lin & Bob Flaws, ISBN 0-936185-24-4

THE DIVINE FARMER'S MATERIA MEDICA (*A Translation of the Shen Nong Ben Cao*) by Yang Shou-zhong ISBN 0-936185-96-1

THE DIVINELY RESPONDING CLASSIC: *A Translation of the Shen Ying Jing from Zhen Jiu Da Cheng*, trans. by Yang Shou-zhong & Liu Feng-ting ISBN 0-936185-55-4

DUI YAO: THE ART OF COMBINING CHINESE HERBAL MEDICINALS by Philippe Sionneau ISBN 0-936185-81-3

ENDOMETRIOSIS, INFERTILITY AND TRADITIONAL CHINESE MEDICINE: A Laywoman's Guide by Bob Flaws ISBN 0-936185-14-7

THE ESSENCE OF LIU FENG-WU'S GYNECOLOGY by Liu Feng-wu, translated by Yang Shou-zhong ISBN 0-936185-88-0

EXTRA TREATISES BASED ON INVESTIGATION & INQUIRY: *A Translation of Zhu Dan-xi's Ge Zhi Yu Lun*, by Yang Shou-zhong & Duan Wu-jin, ISBN 0-936185-53-8

FIRE IN THE VALLEY: TCM Diagnosis & Treatment of Vaginal Diseases ISBN 0-936185-25-2

FLESHING OUT THE BONES: The Importance of Case Histories in Chin. Med. trans. by Chip Chace. ISBN 0-936185-30-9

FU QING-ZHU'S GYNECOLOGY trans. by Yang Shou-zhong and Liu Da-wei, ISBN 0-936185-35-X

FULFILLING THE ESSENCE: A *Handbook of Traditional & Contemporary Treatments for Female Infertility* by Bob Flaws, ISBN 0-936185-48-1

GOLDEN NEEDLE WANG LE-TING: A 20th Century Master's Approach to Acupuncture by Yu Hui-chan and Han Fu-ru, trans. by Shuai Xue-zhong,

A HANDBOOK OF TRADITIONAL CHINESE DERMATOLOGY by Liang Jian-hui, trans. by Zhang & Flaws, ISBN 0-936185-07-4

A HANDBOOK OF TRADITIONAL CHINESE GYNECOLOGY by Zhejiang College of TCM, trans. by Zhang Ting-liang, ISBN 0-936185-06-6 (4th edit.)

A HANDBOOK OF MENSTRUAL DISEASES IN CHINESE MEDICINE by Bob Flaws ISBN 0-936185-82-1

A HANDBOOK of TCM PEDIATRICS by Bob Flaws, ISBN 0-936185-72-4

A HANDBOOK OF TCM UROLOGY & MALE SEXUAL DYSFUNCTION by Anna Lin, OMD, ISBN 0-936185-36-8

THE HEART & ESSENCE OF DAN-XI'S METHODS OF TREATMENT by Xu Dan-xi, trans. by Yang, ISBN 0-926185-49-X

THE HEART TRANSMISSION OF MEDICINE by Liu Yi-ren, trans. by Yang Shou-zhong ISBN 0-936185-83-X

HIGHLIGHTS OF ANCIENT ACUPUNCTURE PRESCRIPTIONS trans. by Wolfe & Crescenz ISBN 0-936185-23-6

**THE SYSTEMATIC CLASSIC
OF ACUPUNCTURE & MOXI-
BUSTION** (*Jia Yi Jing*) by Huang-fu Mi,
trans. by Yang Shou-zhong & Charles Chace,
ISBN 0-936185-29-5

**THE TAO OF HEALTHY EATING
ACCORDING TO CHINESE MED-
ICINE** by Bob Flaws, ISBN 0-936185-
92-9

**THE TREATMENT OF DISEASE
IN TCM, Vol I: Diseases of the Head
& Face Including Mental/Emotional
Disorders** by Philippe Sionneau & Lü Gang,
ISBN 0-936185-69-4

**THE TREATMENT OF DISEASE
IN TCM, Vol. II: Diseases of the
Eyes, Ears, Nose, & Throat** by Sionneau
& Lü, ISBN 0-936185-69-4

**THE TREATMENT OF DISEASE,
VOL. III: Diseases of the Mouth,
Lips, Tongue, Teeth & Gums**, by
Sionneau & Lü, ISBN 0-936185-79-1

**THE TREATMENT OF DISEASE,
VOL IV: Diseases of the Neck, Shoul-
ders, Back, & Limbs**, by Philippe Sionneau
& Lü Gang, ISBN 0-936185-89-9

**THE TREATMENT OF EXTER-
NAL DISEASES WITH
ACUPUNCTURE & MOXI-
BUSTION** by Yan Cui-lan and Zhu Yun-
long, ISBN 0-936185-80-5